Mastering the Art of Taijiquan

Other Titles by the Author

Audacity of Poetry,
Healing in a Word,
With Poetry in Mind,
This is Our Word,
There is Only Music Brother,
Doors to Ancient poetical Echoes,
Lovers Should Never Quarrel,
The Song of Life,
Calm is the Water, and
The Healer Within Us.

Mastering the Art of Taijiquan

Insights into the Path, the Practice,
the Patience, and the Art

Master George E. Samuels

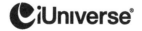

MASTERING THE ART OF TAIJIQUAN
INSIGHTS INTO THE PATH, THE PRACTICE, THE PATIENCE, AND THE ART

iUniverse books may be ordered through booksellers or by contacting:

iUniverse
1663 Liberty Drive
Bloomington, IN 47403
www.iuniverse.com
1-800-Authors (1-800-288-4677)

ISBN: 978-1-4917-6584-5 (sc)
ISBN: 978-1-4917-6585-2 (e)

Library of Congress Control Number: 2015906019

Print information available on the last page.

iUniverse rev. date: 04/28/2015

Contents

Dedication

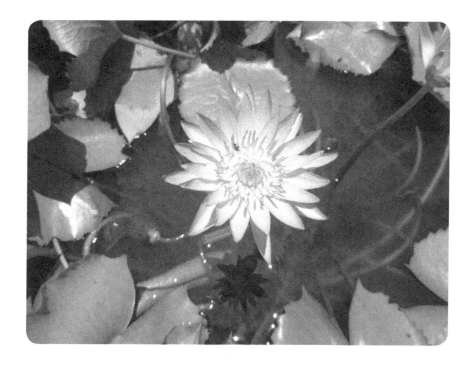

To the Supreme Most High
And
To My Family whether they may be!
Qi
"The end purpose of these energies is to prolong life and endow
it with the youth of eternal spring"(Classic of Taijiquan)

Acknowledgements

To the Ancient Masters who came before to share their knowledge and wisdom

Special Acknowledgement To Master Siu-Fong Evans for help editing, providing insight and understanding including the Chinese characters and proper translations

Special Acknowledgement to Master Chen Song-Tso who openly shares his wisdom with his students

To Grand Master Yun Yin Sen my Liu He Ba Fa Teacher who shared his knowledge and family of friends in Shanghai

To Grand Master Lui Bao Yu my Quan You Teacher who shares his knowledge and wisdom with me

To the numerous Chen Style Masters such as Grandmasters Chen Zhenglei and Chen XiaoWang and many others that helped inspire me to learn Chen Style Taiji

To Master George Xu who tirelessly teaches and shares his higher level skills with others

To all the other Masters and Teachers who honestly share their knowledge and wisdom too numerous to name

To my brother Master Golden Li in Hong Kong and sister Ling Gao who helps all who come to learn

To all the brothers and sisters of the Internal Martial Arts who practice hoping to reach perfection too numerous to name here

Introduction

Taiji is one of the internal martial arts and is practiced by millions around the world. There are many Taiji Masters too numerous to count in China and throughout Asia. Fortunately there are a few masters and teachers who have relocated to different parts of the world such as America, and Europe. *Mastering The Art of Taijiquan* is written to help all those who having practiced Taiji and are trying to become masters of the Art. It sounds simple but in order to become a master, practitioners need a Teacher who has mastered the art, and can share his knowledge and wisdom with those trying to reach the same level. Even with a Teacher one needs to do research on the classics in order to understand the principles until one can replicate them in their practice. Many teachers expect one to do their own research and many students are just led to a certain point and must decipher the rest on their own.

Writing *Mastering the Art of Taijiquan* tries to fill in the blanks for all those practitioners who have no teacher or master, those who are trying to self teach themselves and those who have teachers that have not yet reached the level of masters of the art. The need for this book is predicated on the fact that Taiji and internal martial arts is a gigantic body of knowledge and requires training, research, understanding, a qualified teacher and a lifetime of practice and patience. *Mastering the Art of Taijiquan* also realizes that there are a group of practitioners that are trying to reach higher levels of the art and need assistance, information and insight in order to progress to the next level. Also, *Mastering the Art of Taijiquan* requires one to study a multitude of materials, some old some new in order to learn what is required to become a master of the art. *Mastering the Art of Taijiquan* also was written in order for practitioners to understand that learning and practicing Taiji and internal martial arts as an ART. And one goes through a transformation of consciousness with the goal in mind of progressing and evolving to the level of mastery and high art, not just as a health exercise or self-defense course. It is not easy to meet high level Masters who practice the art of Taiji as an art but in order to spur excellence and evolution of the art in the West, one must understand that Taiji is an art. One must also take the initiative to grow, evolve, elevate their consciousness and gain mastery in the art of Taijiquan.

Mastering the Art of Taijiquan also is written to help those who after practicing, trying to excel, and progress are missing vital information on how to progress to higher levels and correct their forms and practice. This is due to the secrecy of the art and its protection by its Masters and practitioners. Also Taiji is considered a secret art and there is a lot of confusion around what is shared and not shared amongst its practitioners who have paid the price to learn this precious art and treasure and should be served meat and not the milk. But this is part of the confusion because many practitioners overlook the secrets in plain sight, namely the classics that are available for all to see. So *Mastering the Art of Taijiquan* pushes these classics to the forefront and lets practitioners know the secrets are in the classics and the answers to their questions are in the classics. This is why it is imperative to clarify any confusion and misinformation. This is why one must look to the classics just as one looks to the Teacher. Unfortunately most practitioners in the West cannot have the best teachers but that is no excuse, and no reason why all the lovers of the art cannot reach a high level. One should research, study this book directs them to where the answers are located in order to help the practitioners evolve and grow for the Art's sake.

So writing this book is an attempt to foster more teachers and masters, to share vital information with its practitioners and lovers of the art.

Also, this book brings some important classic information together to assist all the practitioners who do not have a teacher teaching explaining the essential points of Taiji that are required, needed and absorbed in order to self-cultivate their mind, body and energy, and transform to a higher level of expertise.

Mastering the Art of Taijiquan is an opportunity to enlighten others to appreciate the art and become lovers of the art. *Mastering the Art of Taijiquan* also answers questions such as, what you need to know to learn and practice Taiji, and other internal gongfu styles as a martial art. Mastering the Art of Taijiquan answers the question; is martial arts only learned for fighting, is that the ultimate goal for internal martial art? *Mastering the Art of Taijiquan* answers the question what is the highest goal of martial arts and Taijiquan? These questions need to be answered so one can channel their ship to the distant shore for arts' sake or for mastery. Renowned Taiji Master Cheng Man Ching stated: "To share good things with others is my true heart's desire." Delve in and enjoy for as we enter the door, we are in a place for artists for arts' sake! Remember Taijiquan is an ultimate art and we must learn as much as we can in order to excel and not be satisfied with low skills. We must seek the high mountain, the consciousness and the wisdom of the art of Taijiquan!

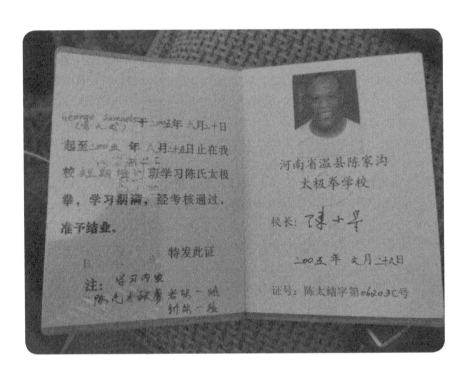

Author Practicing Taiji Jian

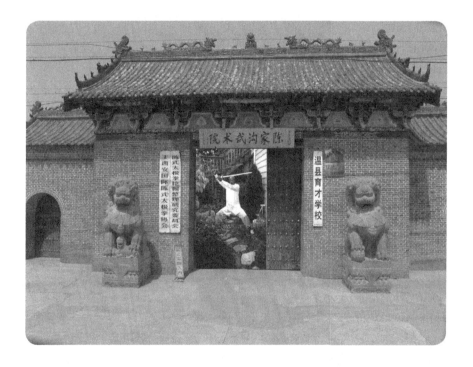

Taiji

Taiji
Up down
Front back
Left right
Circulate the will
Avoid the might
Stand tall
So you can't fall
Feet touching the ball
So the sun can shine on all

Middle of the way
I stand
As night turns to day
Yin opposes yang
As yang chases yin
And all is family
After the kin
Has separated from Wuji
Losing in order to win
Taiji from Wuji

The world from the universe
Heaven and earth
Does not separate
From us
Because we are one
With the universe
Qi, Root and centered
Circulating in unison
All in one breath
From Taiji to back to Wuji.

I

THE PATH

Small Group practicing Taiji

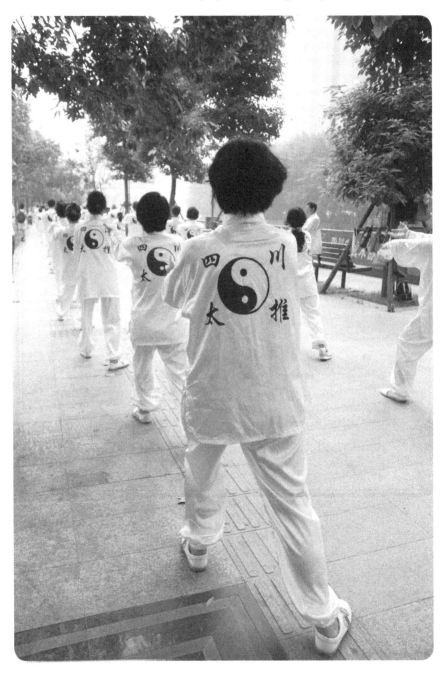

Taiji: What Is It?

Taiji Chuan (Tai Chi Chuan) or Taijiquan, or sometimes, called Taiji or Tai Chi, is a type of internal Chinese martial art practiced for both self defense training and health benefits. There are many versions of Taiji but it is all considered the same. The terms can be used to substitute each other but for this treatise I will try to keep it consistent. We may use any version of Taiji but they will all mean the same and are interchangeable. This is also the same for Qi (energy), which is also called Chi (energy), both means the same. We will cover some basic information and knowledge about Taiji just as we will cover learned lessons, principles, and insights in order to help all those reading this material to benefit from it on some rudimentary, and higher levels. In order to write about Taiji most practitioners, and many Masters wait their whole lifetime to impart some of their immense knowledge or neglect to impart any. Taiji is so deep, and complex, it is important to glean what knowledge, information, insights, or wisdom pearls that are garnered by its practitioners. We can all learn from each other if we are willing to share what we have researched or know from our own individual practices.

Many practitioners want to become masters of the art, is the reason for the importance of sharing valuable information, and insights on the journey to mastering the art. Remember Taijiquan is an art, and we should practice it for Art's sake. I did not write this to dispute or argue what, and who or which forms are better or best or to contradict anyone else. This book is written in order for us to share knowledge, insights, and experiences with each other, as we are all practitioners. All the principles are the same no matter what style you study or practice. We are fortunate that Taiji has a long and generous history to draw upon for us to build our own knowledge base. Taijiquan is China's treasure that is being shared with the world, and we should take full advantage to learn, and enjoy its many benefits! Some of this information is already known, and/or repeated but again remember Taiji's rich history, and the Chinese culture where it was created realizes we are its students, inheritors and benefactors. So let us begin.

Taijiquan is also called "Supreme Ultimate Fist". It is part of the overall Wushu Family. It is practiced differently than external Wushu practice. External Wushu movements are practiced fast, and with force most of the time whereas Taijiquan is practiced slow, and with a minimum of external force but instead utilizes internal power. Taiji has its hard, and soft varieties but is considered an internal martial art. It is important to know what is the difference between external, and internal gongfu forms, and practices. This doesn't mean that Taiji is not practiced fast at the more advanced levels but that it's foundational training requires slow, relaxed, and the minimal use of force. As long as this is adhered to the practitioner trainee is beginning on the right path. Chang quan its wushu equivalent is similar to Taiji except it is an external form practiced at a fast speed.

Attributes of Taijiquan

The attributes of Taijiquan vary from traditional Wushu practice because of the following such as:

- **Softness versus Hardness:** Taijiquan is based on softness but the softness is outside and the hardness is inside. This is why they say Taiji is steel wrapped in cotton, but it is not so soft it is like a wet noodle.
- **Relaxation**: All movements are to be performed with minimum muscle tension. Only enough muscle activity is used to keep the correct posture, and execute the desired gesture. This is an imperative, and one must understand that when you think you are relaxed, relax more.
- **Slowness**: Taiji is about becoming self-aware, the slower you make the movements the more you become aware of the subtle

changes within the body as you pass through a gesture. It will also help you become aware of the "inner workings" of Taiji. It is also said to facilitate the development of "internal power", or nèijìn (内劲).

- **Coordination**: Though different styles may have differing philosophies on how this is achieved, the general consensus is that the art of Taiji develops a body that is working in harmony with itself as one unit.
- **Mindfulness**: The Taiji form should be practiced with mental intent awareness of each phase of the movements. The quieter the mind the better you can be aware of the internal working of Taiji, and the better you can facilitate the mind, body, and spirit integration.
- **Breathing**: Is the link that ties everything together, the emphasis is on deep, natural breathing often referred to as "abdominal breathing". There are many styles that emphasize more sophisticated methods of breathing but breathing natural is best.
- **Circle**: You become the ball and circulate within the circle within the square, which will then create spirals.
- **Invisible**: Internal is invisible; is the practice, and visible is the application.
- **Art**: Taiji is an internal art, remember the emphasis is on the Art not the fighting as the ultimate goal but the higher qualities that make it an Art for self-cultivation of the mind, body and energy.

What do the Classics say Taiji Is?

First Taiji comes from Wuji, which separated and gave birth to yin and yang, then a thousand different things. Classics also say Taiji is a martial art. Taiji consists of two forms that constitute and encompass heaven and earth and represent the opposites such as yin yang, hot and cold, opening and closing, motion and stillness, soft and hard, up and down, left and right, folding and stretching, visible and invisible, inhalation and exhalation, advance and retreat to name a few. The classics concern with the conditions of how to perform internal martial arts which is different than external martial arts such as to move left one must first go right, when one wants to move up one must move down first. If one wants to expand one must shrink and visa versa. Taiji also embodies the idea of there is motion in stillness and stillness in motion along with the idea that for every action there is a reaction and visa versa which is difficult for some to understand and perform. One can say being empty or full but it is important to be able to perform these operations. Using mind and energy instead of muscles and brute strength is for some difficult to understand but essential in Taiji.

So this idea of using the internal as gongfu instead of the external takes a lot to understand, perform, and redevelop how to perform internal martial arts. It takes time, alas the slow movement and slow developmental process in order to master the art. The classics say that even the names they gave the forms give clues to the martial art implied and how to apply them but must be practiced with the idea of the internal practice in mind (a key word). The idea or philosophy of Taijiquan is considered a secret because one must understand consciousness and how it interacts with yourself and the consciousness of others in order to progress and play at a high level. The secrets are revealed though, as you learn and practice the art.

Insight

Understanding all of this requires us to focus on how to learn and master this incredible art. Some may think it is easy but that is only learning the form not the art. So many practitioners after learning the forms realize there is more to learn. I learned this and once knowing this those interested in learning and progressing to a high level must either, have a good teacher or master, and perseverance. I realized later on what was missing is the clear understanding of the expansiveness of the Taiji system and the need to understand the classic principles and a highly qualified Teacher who would share their knowledge and wisdom with their students.

Let's understand Taiji is an internal martial arts practice using the heart and mind to increase and move the Qi, and will increase the flexibility of the body. Taiji training focuses on turning stiffness into softness and back into hardness. At the same time it replaces physical strength into internal strength (force). {刚柔相济: couple hardness and softness to aid each other}

The Qi flows and in turn moves the body from the ground thru the body, which improves the circulation and revitalizes the entire system. It can be used for healing and for self-defense, and to enhance ones' martial art abilities. Taiji encompasses the vital principles of absorbing transforming and directing three forces, which is the forces; from the universal forces, sun, moon, stars, the cosmic forces from the environment, and the earth. Many people spend most of their time on learning and perfecting the forms, outer movements, and don't get to spend the lion's share of time on the internal practice, which is required. The internal connection with life energy is important. The art of Taijiquan is a lot to learn, absorb, and master. This and much more will be discussed later on in subsequent chapters.

Shaolin Kungfu

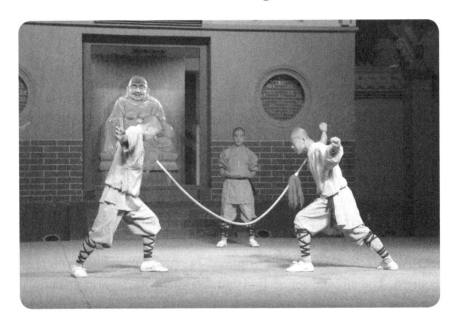

Wushu: A Rich Heritage

Wushu is a cultural and rich heritage of the Chinese people. Wushu has appealed to the masses and has helped with the health, safety and welfare of the Chinese people. The origin of wushu can be traced back to prehistoric times and has always been used as a way to develop fighting skills for self defense and for the improvement of general health and fitness. Its history can be traced and in most cases has been documented, and to date has become an international sport spreading around the globe. The chart below is a short chronological history of wushu.

Zhou Dynasty	11century-256BC	Jiaoli (wrestling) was a sport along with archery and chariot racing
Warring States Period	403-221BC	Wushu for the army pointed out in Sunzi (book on the art of war)
Qin Dynasty	221BC-206BC	Growth of fighting arts such as shoubo (wrestling)
Jin Dynasty	420-581	Ge Hong integrated Wushu with Qigong as part of Chinese medicine
Tang Dynasty	618-907	Court examinations and major development of Wushu
Song Dynasty	960-1279	Wushu societies
Ming Dynasty	1368-1644	16 different styles was compiled
Qing Dynasty	1644-1911	Taiji, pigua and eight diagram schools established
Peoples Republic	1949-	Much has been done and continues to promote Wushu, and Chinese culture and Wushu has spread around the globe

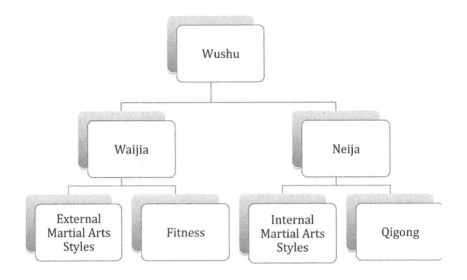

External or Internal Martial Art

Wushu (called kungfu or gongfu in the West) is a form of martial art that is practiced for training the body, and for self-defense. The basic methods of wushu are considered external in practice and, focus on training the body to become a weapon. External wushu mainly focuses on physical strength (Li) as the significant point of power. Taiji and all internal wushu forms differ and are the same because they mainly focus on energy as the main point of power. Both hard and soft wushu of which Taiji and all internal forms are a part of focus on skills, and techniques but external forms can be seen and expressed externally. All internal forms such as Taiji also focuses on skills, and techniques but are expressed internally before being expressed externally which makes the appearance to be considered invisible to the naked untrained eye.

Wushu is divided into categories that separate the external from the internal arts branches. The external branches are known as waijia and the internal branches are known as neijia (Nèi jiā quán 内家拳.) The wushu branches are clearly divided in order to understand the principles of each, and the main focus can be broken into branches from the same tree. *Mastering the Art of Taijiquan* will focus on the internal branches of Taijiquan but one must include the internal principles and the importance of Qigong, which belongs to the same branch of neijia (neigong.)

Neigong

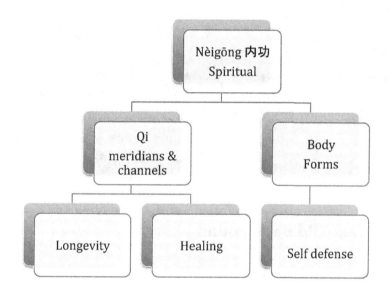

Neigong Practice

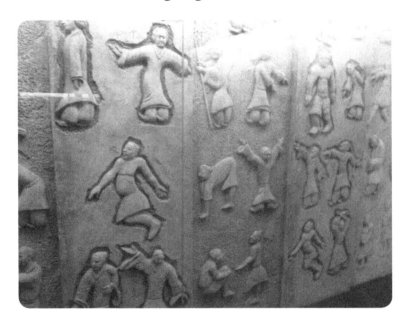

5000-Year-Old Background

Neigong内功 (neigung):

Is it an internal exercise or skill? Neigong includes Qigong breathing exercises, loosening exercises (daoyin) and different forms of energy (Jin) exercises. Neigong is in many respects the Chinese equivalent of the Indian yoga system. Neigong originated in the Chinese philosophy of the Dao, the religion of Taoism (Daoism), Traditional Chinese Medicine and folklore, and has a 5000-year history. Neigong is a part of the daoist Neidan practice of internal alchemy.

Neigong: (Daoyin Exercises)

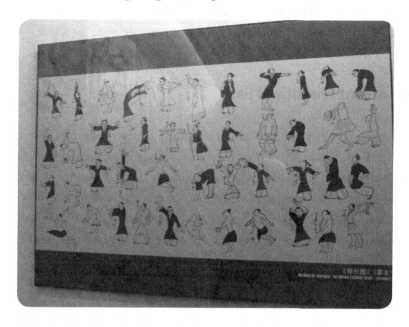

There are a great number of different exercises, which cultivates the treasures of Jing (Essence), Qi (Chi, energy, air, breath or life force) and Shen (Spirit) for health, longevity and enlightenment. Here are a few examples of groups of neigong exercises:

- **Standing meditation** (Standing like a tree, Standing Pole or Standing Post) in Chinese Zhanzhuang or San Ti,
- **Different forms of meditation** (dantian Yi Sou Dan Tien, small circulation Shao Chou Tien or grand circulation Da Chou Tien),
- **Breathing techniques** (prenatal breathing, moving and still forms of Qigong (Qikung) as Baduanjin (Eight Pieces of Brocade), Tortoise
- **Walking meditation** (Kinhin),
- **Different forms of massage therapy** (Tuina, Shiatzu, acupressure)
- **Body tapping of meridians**, acupoint and body parts (upper, middle and lower dantian).

Food, herbs, diet therapy and parts of Traditional Chinese Medicine are also included as part of prevention of sickness, healing and theory of longevity, which is also a part of the esoteric neigong practice.

Important Historical Fact

Everyone can see external wushu forms quite clearly. All forms of wushu are utilized for a variety of reasons such as self-defense, healing, training, fortifying the body, longevity, demonstrations and competitions. Within the body of wushu practices whether they are waijia or neijia, they are broken down into two main categories, called traditional and modern or contemporary wushu. Taiji has the same history as wushu when it comes to the traditional versus the contemporary.

These two methods, one traditional with a long, true and tried history behind them and, the second is considered modern or contemporary styles which have a short, condensed history but are taken from the traditional methodology. The training is quite different but considered to provide a supposedly similar result, which is up for debate. Internal, and external training of wushu are trained and practiced differently because external forms are taught and practiced at a faster speed to develop speed, strength, and power whereas the internal forms are trained, and practiced at a slow speed in order to build energy, and internal power. Both types of wushu will build health but the idea of soft versus hard techniques separate the two. It should also be noted here that, at this stage, the art that was to become known as Taijiquan was originally considered to be Chang quan or Long Fist Boxing before soft methodologies was added.

Even though there are a multitude of styles within the Taiji schools there are six or seven traditional main schools: Chen, Yang, Wu (Hao), Wu, Sun and Wudang. There are many more such as Li and Fu styles to name a few. These are all branches of the same tree, and contribute to the rich body of knowledge of Taijiquan. These schools can be further condensed into two traditional schools of philosophy called Buddhist or Daoist traditions. The modern or contemporary schools of forms differ because one, they stem from the University, Chinese Sports Commission and were essentially created for competitions, and two some Taiji Masters recreated forms to make it easy for the masses to learn or that is what they say. Other modern condensed forms such as the Yang, WU and Chen style forms are created to assist those in learning from short routines that can be utilized to teach a broad base of practitioners around the world.

Listed below are five most recognized styles of Taiji. I added Wudang, which is growing rapidly. There are many more but these are the most well known:

- Chen 陈式
- Yang 杨式
- Wu Hao 武式
- Sun 孙式
- Wu 吴式
- Wudang 武当

Insight

It is important to clarify that there is a difference between the traditional and the modern Taijiquan forms. Including the way it is taught and practiced so one can conform to its requirements. The principles are supposed to be the same but most of the time in modern style Taiji; forms are practiced in order to provide a vehicle for basic health and for competitions.

So one must understand as they practice the requirements for example, in the modern style when practicing the postures one must look and fulfill the standards for competitions whereas when practicing the traditional way the internal expression is paramount, and the focus is not solely on the presentation that will garner one with a gold medal or trophy. The focus is on the principles and so it does not matter the length of the form but the focus on the principles adhered as one practices the forms.

Taiji Group Performance

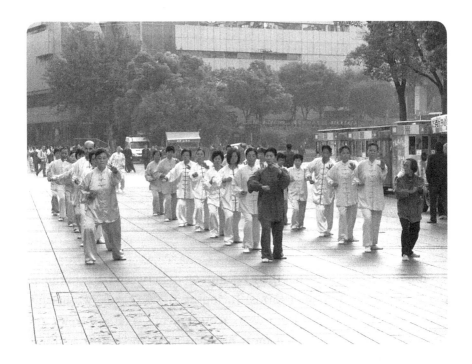

Origins

I will not get involved with who or what came first the chicken or the egg but there are two schools of thought. The first is that Taiji was developed and practiced in the early 1800's in a place called Chenjiagou affectionately known as Chen Village and Zhaobao Town. The second is that Taiji was developed and practiced at Wudang in the 12th century by a Taoist monk called Zhang Sanfeng. (Zhang Sanfeng may or may not be a legendary figure, some say there is no proof.) That is why The Chen family claimed it is their ancestor Chen Wang Ting that created Taijiquan. When Chen Wang Ting retired, records say he created quanshu. There is proof that this may be so. There is a lot of research about this but we won't concern ourselves with that and let others more versed in history to contemplate that. There are many styles of Taijiquan but they all were derived from Chen Style Taiji. We will focus on the Art of Taiji and internal martial arts because all styles utilize similar principles at the higher level. It is not the style that matters but the art and we are here to gain as much knowledge as we can garner.

Both Chenjiagou and Wudang like Shaolin have a wealth of knowledge, and skills and are considered part of the main centers of Taiji practice, and philosophy. Both have a rich history of the Art so they can both share the glory in my eyes. If you really want to know more visit both in China, and there you can discuss the development of the art of wushu, and Taiji. I have visited both Chenjiagou and Wudang and happy that I was fortunate to be able to. Taijiquan is an authentic living Chinese treasure that is being practiced now around the world.

Taijiquan Lineage Tree

To better understand Taiji and other internal arts one should view and research various lineage. There are many lineage trees for all the

Taijiquan styles, which are long and serve us well if we want to know, and understand the history but the object of *Mastering The Art of Taijiquan* is to provide in-depth insight into the mastering of Taijiquan. China has patiently protected its history, and lineage by documenting it for us to understand its ancestral families, Masters, disciples, and Teachers. **You can access the lineage of individual styles when you do your research.** Taiji is reaching around the globe and its practitioners are growing so the lineage will continue to grow.

Beginning Historical Overview

Taijiquan is a branch of the traditional internal martial arts (or Nei Jia Kung Fu) that spread widely in China over 300 years ago at the beginning of the Qing Dynasty. It became very popular starting around 1911 in Beijing. Stories abound about how this martial art we call Taijiquan, may have developed around the eighth century.

Nei Jia (Internal Shape) Kung Fu is a term that has became associated with the grouping of Internal Chinese Martial Arts known more generally as: Baguazhang (Eight Diagrams Palm), Xingyiquan (Form and Will Boxing), and Taijiquan (Supreme Ultimate Fist). All three of these arts are known for their health maintenance properties and their sophisticated approach to self-defense that is generally characterized by seeking softness, patience and flexibility over hardness, speed and brute force. This approach is different from Wai (External) Jia Martial Arts, which are characterized by maximizing speed and physical force. A well-known example of Wai Jia is Shaolin (and the multitude of styles and variations that it includes). In this context, a person can practice Taijiquan, for example, and refer to them self as a practitioner of Nei Jia Kung Fu. Each of these arts is a complete martial arts system.

In the beginning wushu was utilized for self-defense to protect its citizens from bandits and others meaning harm to families, and their communities or villages. Wushu was also used to protect soldiers from local, and foreign invaders. Wushu also provided an added benefit by making its practitioners more healthy, and fit. By realizing this health benefit wushu was taught to the infirm as a way of making them healthy, and providing benefits of longevity. By the same token some of the practitioners of wushu used their skills to rob, and take advantage of those less powerful. This caused a great problem especially amongst the more fragile or peaceful population such as farmers, and those not trained or engaged in warlike behavior. The wushu practitioners were so powerful that it required a different methodology in order to contend with them, in order to subdue them, and protect the innocent families especially living in the more suburban, and rural areas.

When dealing with strong individuals there is a "might meets might" clause that is met, and the winner is normally attributed to who is the strongest. Those not that powerful needed to realize that strength versus strength wasn't going to serve them, and they needed something more substantial such as skills, and techniques to protect their families and communities. Whoever discovered it first paved the way for genius to arise, and show that the path to success was to not pit strength against strength but to pit strength against skills, and techniques in order to win, and keep the families safe from strong, powerful warlords and robbers. Thus we begin to understand the wisdom of the Taiji Ages.

Paths of Taiji

The path of Taiji and other internal martial arts is varied so one must choose what is their individual goal(s) and then focus on it. It is up to the individual to choose and enjoy their practice of the art of Taiji. But lets be clear so there is no confusion in the future thinking you were training for one goal and ended up on another track or path and didn't realize it. Below we outline the paths, some will be duel paths but at least we are clear and focused.

○ *For health*
Practice only for health, to improve one's health and ward off sickness

○ *For performance or competition*
Win many medals and trophies and become a grand champion

○ *For self defense*
Learn how to use the art of Taiji to defend myself

○ *For mastery*
Master the forms and learn to use Taiji for health and self-defense, push hands utilizing internal skills such as Dong Jin and Ling Kong Jin

○ *For high art*
Practice as an integral part of my daily regimen, learn the forms, the applications, how to use the art to help and heal myself, and others by sharing my skill and knowledge and practice for art's sake. For the cultivation of higher consciousness.

○ *For combat*
Using Taiji for pure combat requires combat training to prepare the body for fighting. This is quite different then basic self-defense, it also requires learning pushing hands for fighting.

Insight: Why Practice Taijiquan?

Yes, ask yourself why are you practicing Taijiquan instead of the litany of wushu external and different internal styles. Is it for fighting or the cultivation of energy or consciousness? Are you serious and if you are there are a lot of brothers and sisters who love and practice the art of Taiji. There are a lot of styles and we can choose whichever one(s) we prefer. It is important to get a teacher if at all possible because no book or DVD can take the place of a highly qualified teacher who is willing to share his knowledge and wisdom. Once you know why you are practicing, do the art well. It is important to study Chinese culture at the same time because it is intertwined within the art of Chinese Wushu, external and internal. I have learned that it is important to start at the history and build a solid foundation in the beginning. Taiji is a science and philosophy so one must read and study alongside their practice.

Basic Foundational Knowledge is Historical

Trigrams

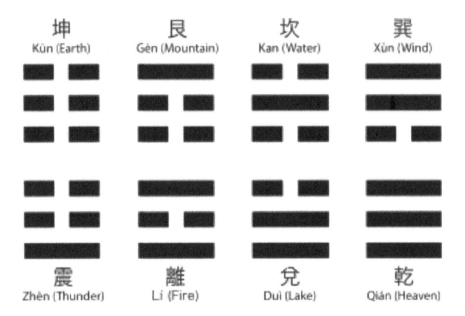

(The eight trigrams

The solid line represents yang, the creative principle. The open line represents yin, the receptive principle. These principles are also represented in a common circular symbol (☯), known as Taijitu (太極圖), but more commonly known in the west as the yin-yang (陰陽) diagram, expressing the idea of complementarity of changes: when Yang is at top, Yin is increasing, and vice versa. For more information research the full Yi Jing.)

Basic foundational knowledge such as the Yi Jing, the Yellow Emperor's Classic of Internal Medicine, the Dao De Jing (Tao te Ching) by Lao Tzu are helpful in understanding the practice of internal martial arts forms such as Taiji since the foundational structure was derived from these ancient cultural philosophies. We will cover them as an overview in order to understand the foundation of Taijiquan. Lao Tzu stated that "water is the softest but can penetrate mountains and the earth, this clearly shows the principle of softness can overcome hardness."

Yi Jing （易经）

Yi Jing also known as the Book of Changes is one of the oldest text containing a divination system of philosophy and cosmology intrinsic to Chinese culture. It centered on the ideas of the dynamic balance of opposites, the evolution of events as a process, and acceptance of the inevitability of change. The system has been developed into 64 sets of 6 called hexagrams representing yin or yang (broken lines or solid lines which are representing yang). Within the 64 hexagrams there are eight trigrams expressed by an arrangement of broken and solid lines that are created to represent the different aspects of life from the directions of west, east, north and south; animals; relationships; binary values; images of nature; states of mind and being and etc.

The Yi Jing connection to Taiji is expressed in the practical exercises as they pertain to the philosophical context of Taoism. This is a reflective, mystical Chinese tradition first associated with the scholar and mystic Lao Tzu, an older contemporary of Confucius. He wrote and taught in the province of Honan in the 6th century B.C. and authored the seminal work of Taoism, the **Tao Te Jing**. As a philosophy, Taoism has many elements but fundamentally it espouses a calm, reflective and mystic view of the world steeped in the beauty and tranquility of nature.

Taiji also has, particularly amongst eastern practitioners, a long connection with the **Yi Jing** a Chinese system of divination. There are associations between the 8 basic Yi Jing trigrams plus the five elements of Chinese alchemy (metal, wood, fire, water and earth) with the thirteen basic postures of Taiji. There are also other associations with the full 64 trigrams of the Yi Jing and other movements in the Taiji forms.

There is no need to rewrite the Yi Jing since there are hundreds of translations of the Yi Jing into English alone, to say nothing of translations and commentaries into almost every language of the world. So you can further research the Yi Jing by reading and studying one of those translations. It's important to notice the connection of the Baqua, which is the circular form of the Yi Jing. The trigrams are related to Taiji philosophy, Taijiquan and the wu xing, or "five elements". The five elements represent wood, earth, air, metal and fire. The Yi Jing focuses on the scientific explanation of creation, Wuji and the birth of yin and yang. It also explains the relationships between Heaven and Earth and the universal including the development of man and his relationship to Heaven and Earth and the universe. This knowledge explains much of the understanding of Taijiquan as the Grand Ultimate Fist.

Baqua

八卦 BaQua

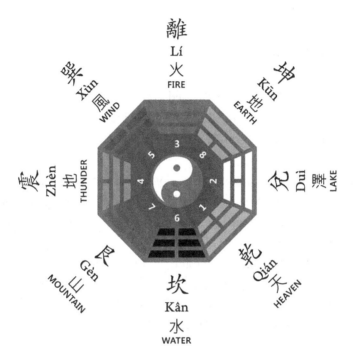

Linking directly to the Taoist principles of the eight trigrams of the Yi Jing and the five elements are the thirteen movements or energies in that include:

Eight postures:

- Ward-off
- Rollback
- Press
- Push
- Pull
- Split
- Elbow strike; and
- Shoulder strike

And five "attitudes" or directions:

- Advance
- Retreat
- Look left
- Gaze right; and

Central equilibrium

The terms for these postures expressed as energies is as follows: 掤、捋、挤、按, 采、挒、肘、靠Peng, Lu, Ji, An, Cai, Lie, Zhou, and Kao are equated to the Eight Trigrams.

The first four are the cardinal directions: Qian (South; Heaven) Kun (North; Earth) Kan [West; Water] Li [East; Fire] The second four are the four corners: Sun [Southwest; Wind] Chen (Northeast; Thunder) Tui (Southeast; Lake) Ken (Northwest; Mountain) Advance (Chin), Withdraw (退Tui) Look Left (顾gu),), Look Right (盼Pan) Central Equilibrium (中定Zhong Ding) are equated to the five elements: Metal, Wood （木mu), Water (水shui), Fire (火huo), and Earth （土tu). All together these are termed the Thirteen Postures.

Attributes of the Five-Element Theory

Direction	Yin organs	Yang Organs	Element	Color
east	liver	Gall bladder	wood	green
west	lungs	Large intestine	metal	white
south	heart	Small intestine	fire	red
north	kidneys	Urinary bladder	water	blue

	Energy Elements			
metal	melt		advance	
wood	expanding		retreat	
water	Gathering, covering		Shift to left	
fire	releasing		Shift to right	
earth	balance	Stomach	center	Golden yellow

Insight

The thirteen postures must be studied and practiced until one is clear as to what they are, how they are performed, and the wisdom of their uses. These postures or energies are learned via the forms so one should be able to recognize them as you learn, and practice the forms. At the same time the five elements should be understood, realizing energies are drawn into the body flowing through from different directions and affect different organs. This helps healing and the fine-tuning of organs especially when you practice Taiji and Qigong. Energy can flow from the earth and also from the Heaven and Universe. Colors also affect the body and its energies.

Understanding The DAO (道Way)

Many people talk about the Dao. The Dao basically means, what is it in the life that we live, and deal with everyday from the universe, the earth, nature, and the flow of things that transpire on a daily basis. We like to think we control everything including the ebb, and flow of the sea, and the wind. These are natural occurrences in which we have little or no control but we only observe, and experience as we walk the earth, and have our being. Our understanding of Taiji should become like the

Dao of which we practice the art just as we move, and have our being each and every day starting with Wuji. (There are ways to interpret the Dao, yet it always goes back to Nature. Buddha has its own way of Dao, Lao Tzu has his own interpretation of Dao...Wuji is part of the Dao at its origin, so there are many interpretations of the Dao.)

Wuji （无极）

Wuji is considered to be the mother of all that represents the Void or beginning before movement was created in the universe. We have all heard the statement that "Wuji is the mother of all and from Wuji sprang everything. Wuji the mother who divided and created yin and yang then the universe sprang forth. That yin, and yang also represents man, and women as we have all passed through the gate of Wuji, from the Mother we have come into being. Above is the heaven and below is the earth. Yang is above in heaven and yin is below in earth. The Light is heaven and the darkness is the earth. In Taiji when we begin we are in a state of Wuji until we step out and separate into yin and yang.

Insight into the Universe

The universe sprang forth in all its glory for man, and women, and all that we have and experience comes from the universal, which presents its self as the Dao that we deal with everyday as it changes, and remains the same day after day. This universal Dao has an effect on each and every one of us, each and everyday throughout our lives. This can be positive or negative or neutral but we are still affected by the Universal Dao changes that occurs in the universe, it nature, and within each of us. For those of us who practice martial arts this affects us, and teaches us that the universe is larger than we realize, as we have much to learn about it, and ourselves as we obtain understanding of external and internal martial arts. What this statement means is that the forces in nature also flow within, and externally, and we must learn to understand them as we learn how to control forces that we intercept, and interact with, including our own internal forces including those of others who we come in contact with during our martial art practices. We are a microcosm of the external (macrocosm) universe, and so represent it even within our practice, and our life.

Insight

This is the basic beginning of the foundation of Taijiquan and should be clearly understood within our practice. As we begin to understand Wuji, then yin and yang, we must start at the beginning, which is important as a foundation in our training. One such vital importance whether we train in external or internal styles is the symbol representing the yin yang. The symbol of yin and yang represents the continual flow and flux of the nature, the universe and Taijiquan. When one is standing still they are in Wuji and when they move they create yin yang. Yin yang is then everywhere in all we do and function. One must clearly understand that. The natural order and flow of nature and the universe represents the Dao.

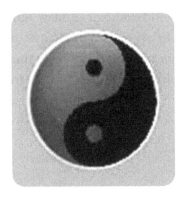

Taiji: Insight into the (Yin/Yang) Symbol

The Yin Yang symbol is a diagram that shows the universe as it is divided from Wuji. The yin yang symbol represents the opposites such as positive and negative, hard and soft, that is expressed in martial arts and Taijiquan. The yin yang symbol also explains Taijiquan when you learn how to reflect soft, hard, left, right, hot, cold, up, down, and front, back in your practice. The yin yang symbol also shows how energy is expressed so that one can understand that even when you express yin, you will express some part of the yang just as when you express yang, you will express some part of the yin at the same time. Included is also the expression of internal versus external.

As a Taijiquan practitioner you must focus on the internal but will also express the external simultaneously. The Yin Yang symbol is very important within your practice, and will be understood when you begin to practice push hands or any applications. This means that before applications one must practice the art of yin yang within the practice of the forms. Once integrated, the yin yang will be evident, and show internally, and externally. Through this practice of yin yang, the energies of the internal practice will be developed, and refined. Since yin and yang are the most important principle one must understand when moving from Wuji what is transpiring. There are examples in the chart below giving a practitioner an understanding of the attributes of the expression of yin yang change.

Yin	Yang
earth	heaven
inhale	exhale
Sinking down	Rising up
contract	expand
close	open
soft	hard
storing	releasing
defense	attack

Insight

As one practices they are always expressing some aspect of yin and yang. If one expresses up, one must also express down, if one expresses left, one must express right, if one expresses forward one will also express backwards, so forth, and so on. Additionally, the circle must be adhered to within the execution of the forms practice. The same will be evident within the push hands practice.

If you don't see or feel any circle or circular movement you are not practicing Taijiquan. If there is no up when there is down or no right when there is left then you are not expressing yin yang in your practice. If it is not clear in your mind yin and yang then you have to research this, and insure you are expressing it within your training. You must know what parts of your body is yin or yang for example if the left leg is yin then the right leg may be yang. If the one arm is yin is the other arm yang? Yin and yang interplay throughout our body and internal system. If you don't sense the yin yang principle you may be double weighted so check. Internally and externally, we are always yin and yang within different parts of our body system.

Internal versus External Expression

This is a dilemma, because many practitioners of Taijiquan get confused about what one may be actually expressing. Is it external only, or is it internal only, or is it a combination of both. To understand this fact many Taiji practitioners in the earlier stages of their practice express the external and if fortunate later express the internal. This is explained much more when we discuss attainment so that a practitioner will understand how to determine where they are in their practice. Many practitioners think they are expressing internal gongfu only to find out their Taijiquan is only the external expression of the form and the art. This is an imperative point that all internal practitioners need to research, understand, and learn to discern in order to assist in their development and the mastery of Taijiquan.

Insight

For example, I may block your punch or your press but am I using my stiff muscle (Li) or am I using Peng (Jin) energy. There is one way (Li) that is external with my strength and the other is internal using Peng jin (energy). You must learn to know the difference, and know which one you are performing and expressing.

There are Other Internal Forms

There are other forms of internal gongfu, which are similar to Taijiquan, they are Baqua and Xingyi and Lui He Ba Fa. All of these internal forms must be understood as internal practices in order to master their art. It is important to note that the same as in the yin yang symbol all internal gongfu art forms also will express external even as they express their dominant internal art. All internal art forms are expressed via the circle, spiral, through the straight line and the square internally and externally.

Movement theory in Baqua is the continuous loop of the circle that is always moving with no end insight. Xingyiquan is expressed via the ever-moving forward straight line, via the circle, never backing up. Taijiquan expresses the circle in the square but within the circle uses the straight line as the diameter or radius utilized within that circle which will create spirals also. Lui He Ba Fa (Water Style Boxing) being a combination of Taiji, Baqua and Xingyi uses the circles and spirals in-combination of the straight moving from the circle and understanding of what's up is down and down is up and the middle ground called Zhong, namely heaven, earth and the middle. This trinity also is representative of man's feet standing on earth and man (head) also connected to the heavens above and to the universe.

Of course, we are all understanding the outward external expression but being internal, the movements are first initiated from the internal before they are witnessed externally. Once this is understood then it has to be dissected to understand how to practice internal boxing such as Taijiquan. This is easily said in an environment where many are learning Taijiquan for health, and competition, which focuses on the external expression or outward appearance of the forms to garner success in the competitive area.

Once the competitions are over then much is required to be understood, including the requirements of internal boxing to adequately practice, and teaching the internal aspects of Taijiquan. Many say they are teaching it but that can be debated as to what they are exactly teaching at a later date. First you must understand the concept of Wushu versus Taijiquan.

Insight

The beginning of the study of Taiji requires one to build and understand the basic foundation so just like a house one must lay a solid foundation of which to build upon in order to build a strong house or practice. If one builds a house on sand it will not have a strong foundation, the same if man builds a house on water it will also move off of its foundation. This is why we cannot miss the opportunity to build a proper foundation in order to build out Taiji practice on.

Insightful Concept of Wushu (Kungfu) versus Taiji

The concept of Wushu versus Taijiquan should be kept to understanding how to learn, and practice with the understanding how one can transverse the bridge from Wushu (external) to (internal) Taijiquan practice. There are similarities, and there are differences. So what are the similarities and differences?

Similar versus Difference

This chart will show some of the differences and similarities of both external and internal. Remember though that in some cases both share the same attributes but are expressed differently. For example both throw punches but they are expressed differently. Wushu throws a focused hard punch, fast to the target to generate power while the Taijiquan punch is relaxed thrown then tensed on impact or can be relaxed on impact using fajin internal force.

Wushu (Kungfu)	Taijiquan
Martial art	Martial art
external	internal
strength	power
muscles	energy
Physical focus (body)	Mind intent
visible	invisible
hard	soft
tense	relax
Block	neutralize
linear	circular

Insight

The wind soft or strong appears, and we all feel and experience it but no one knows where the wind comes from. Wind can be gentle or change and blow your house down. Water flows around the world but no one knows from where it begins. They just know its passes by their way. Water can be gentle or a wave can knock you down and can also allow you to sink into it covering you totally. Yet it can float your boat.

The Basic Understanding

This primary understanding of internal boxing is required in order to begin to create the foundation of the internal practice:

- If you don't understand the hard you won't understand the soft.
- If you don't understand the difference between external and internal you won't understand the internal, and you will practice the internal the same as one will practice the external.
- If you don't understand Qi you won't understand internal movement

This will cause one not to progress to the level of internal practitioner mastery. Once you understand the basic difference then you can begin to train with the understanding that you are not learning an external martial art, but an internal one even if you have already learned the external postures first. Think of it like you are going to school with the mindset you will go to college, or instead of further training (education) your goal is only to go to school, get a high school diploma and then just find a job.

So with this understanding you can decide if you are going to just practice for health, or learn to compete or go on to accomplish the highest level. Once clear begin the process of training and completing the developmental steps it takes to master the internal art of Taijiquan.

Overview of the Levels of Attainment in the Practice of Taijiquan

When I first finished my first form (Yang Style 24 form) the instructor said that he was done and all we had to do was practice it and maybe in 25 years we may get something or not. I was concerned because I had a background in karate and I know this could not be it. I took a trip to Beijing and saw high level practitioners who explained that one needs more than just practicing 25 years and hope you get something or not. As I found and met other Teachers from Chen Village who taught the Chen style Taiji, I knew this was better for me to study because it was more traditional. It had numerous postures that were varied and generated some martial aspects that were easily discernible. I practiced sincerely and eventually I entered into several competitions and won several medals. Afterwards, I still felt something was still lacking, so I searched and when I met a high level Taiji Master, he explained that I had only learned the external part of the Taiji forms, which was great for competition but I needed to continue my study, and practice the internal gongfu methods of the Taiji. Additionally, he explained that there are several levels all trainees, and practitioners should be aware of so that we won't mistakenly think once we master the forms that we are at the end of our journey and journey to mastery.

The major levels or as I call them the three steps of the Taiji ladder of gongfu; first level are lian xi 练习, which refers to the development and practice of the postures and their techniques. The second is developing Dong Jin 懂劲, which implies that you have practiced the forms, and not only know the postures but the function and have developed the eight jins and have mastered the principles of Taiji. The third level is shen ming 神明 which is the level of enlightenment and cultivation whereby you have experienced the treasures of the art of Taiji and you now practice for the spiritual enlightenment and the cultivation of higher consciousness. Understanding the major levels we then can move forward with our practice to train, progress and accomplish the levels until we reach that high level of mastery.

What are the levels of progression? The levels of training constitute how we begin to train with the understanding that at first we train the physical doing the basic gongfu movements. Many martial art practices have levels of progression and some have belt structures, which in Taiji or internal Wushu are unnecessary except to hold up your pants. As we practice, and go through the training from our Instructors, we continue to do the physical requirements, which we call foundational but at the same time we should begin to learn how to train, and practice using the internal requirements because Taiji is an internal art.

As we grow in our internal training, and understanding we rely less on the physical, and one moves toward the internal practice to our goal of internal martial arts practitioner until we reach the level of Internal Master. This is a long path that requires practice, and dedication but can be reached if we stay true to our goal. The chart shows you what is your emphasis beginning with the physical, and the use of the internal. When you reach the level of mastery you will then express the internal through the external but all focus will start from the internal, and will be essentially be invisible until it is expressed. The levels are a natural progression as you grow in your practice. We can write a book about each level but it is just as important to know there are levels, and ponder where we are as we practice. A qualified Taijiquan Teacher will know when you have progressed to the next level. These levels are not set in stone and they are known and I added a couple of my own opinion also. This helps to clear up the misconceptions some have as to where they are or how to gauge their progression in their practice.

Levels	External	Internal	Training
Level one	90	10	foundational
Level two	80	20	structural
Level three	70	30	energetic

Level four	60	40	intentional
Level five	50	50	Combination meta-physical
Level six	40	60	Purely Internal
Level seven	30	70	Spiritual enlightenment

Insight

Why are the levels of training necessary? So one is clear because as we complete the curriculum we are clear as to how we have progressed. The curriculum is; basic foundation training, empty hand forms training, push hands training, weapons training and combat training. We don't have to give you a color belt to let you know what level you are or where you have progressed even though some western teachers feel the need. Traditional Masters gave no such belt but the levels are only to help you with understanding the amount of external to internal one is practicing so you can adjust your practice in a way that leads you to higher, and deeper training while you are learning, and refining your internal practice. This will only assist your understanding, and provide a gauge so you can stay on course, and strive higher.

Some practitioners stay at the first or second level, and that is ok if that is your goal. Other practitioner deepen their practice, and go on to higher levels because they have different goals while others just want to know how to strive, and get to the next level of their practice to becoming Taiji Masters of the Art of Taijiquan. The next question is how do we get to the next step. One way is to study the Classics. Without the Classics the journey is arduous. So let us begin with the Song of Taiji.

The Song of Taiji

"The source of life is at the waist.
Pay attention to 'apparent' and 'solid', Without hindrance Qi flows with grace.
Stillness in movement, movement in stillness, Adjust according to what the situation is.
Every move most be guided by will. Combat efficiency will be achieved with ease.
All the time pay attention to your waist, The abdomen is charged with Qi and might.
The spine is straight and full of spirit; The whole body is relaxed with the head upright.
Be attentive to the details in every move, Spontaneous let your movements be.
A teachers' guidance is needed to enter the way, When accomplished, unrestricted by the rules are you.
What is so difficult about the form? Mind and energy are the king.
What is the aim of Taijiquan practice? Health and vitality and the eternal spring."

Insight

This Classic Song of Taiji begins to point the way, and it is not to be taken lightly but should be garnered as pearls, and just as valuable. Think about what you are reading and internalize it slowly as you continue your practice. Some classics you read may duplicate what you already know or not know. So, therefore one should absorb these words slowly knowing you will be able to reach this goal in the future. Remember, "Mind and energy are King", this is most important for all internal practitioners. Think about what you are paying attention to!

GrandMaster Chen Zhenglei and the Author

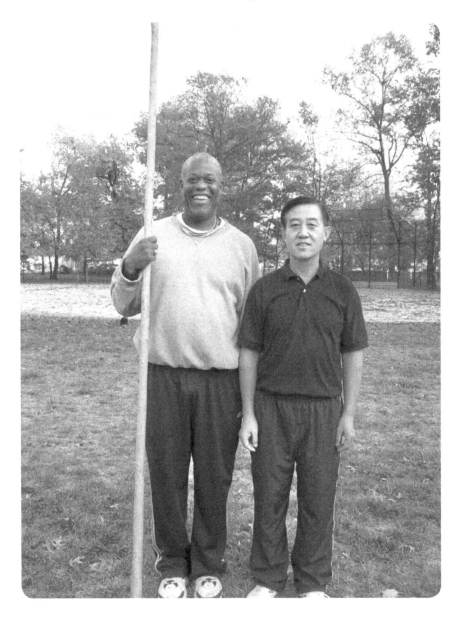

Taiji Quan versus Taiji Gong

This is important to discuss and understand because there is a difference between the two. Quan means fist and gong means skill and energy. Many practitioners learn Taijiquan. Few learn Taijigong (kung). The difference between quan (forms) training, and gong (kung) training is that gong means one is developing and cultivating energy. When one learns Taiji they will need to know which one they are learning. Both are vital and essential training but knowledge of what is the your individual goal, and what is the goal of the Teacher is important. If this is known in advance then it is easy to distinguish the difference, then both the teacher and the student is in harmony and there is no confusion. If you want to learn gong training and your Teacher doesn't teach that it's important you realize this so you can decide if you want to practice gong or understand what to do once you have learned the quan part of your training. Some Teachers can teach both and are willing to teach both and some other Teachers only teach quan which ok. Once you have learned the quan you can seek a Teacher to learn the gong. Energy cultivation is an integral part of Taiji and if you don't learn and practice gong you will not be able to reach a higher level in the art of Taiji.

Insight

The importance of learning and understanding both quan and gong is like two sides of a coin. One side doesn't make a coin only half of a coin so those who want to be masters must include both sides of the coin, quan and gong. The mastery of Taiji requires both and it is just a matter of when you learn. If you feel you want to master the art of Taiji then you will need to incorporate both into your practice. Remember qigong and neigong are the heart of Taijiquan.

Insights from My Personal Journey

I practiced Taiji for more then 20 years off and on with a variety of Teachers, learning a variety of forms. I attended lots of workshops and seminars on a variety of subjects. All of this helped me and I was enthusiastic about learning but found many of the teachers were either not Masters of the art, external Wushu (武术)masters and teachers, or were lacking certain aspects that I felt was missing. One of those elements was the foundational training besides just a basic warm up. The other was functionality. The forms appeared to be empty and the training of the forms was ok but there didn't appear to be any growth beyond learning and practicing the external postures. Prevalent was the idea that there were secrets, and some people received information while others was denied. I didn't understand this since many people had spent their hard earned funds to learn, I felt this was a problem. Sharing of information by a teacher should be to help students to grow not stunt their growth. For the lovers of the art of Chinese martial arts it is disingenuous to give them a little and leave out the most important aspects of the art, and it is a shame. It is a shame because these people are in most cases genuine practitioners of the art and are representative of this Chinese treasure, the art of internal martial arts. I witnessed that this turned off many would be practitioners and lovers of Chinese internal martial arts who quit and turned to Karate because their teacher either taught only the form, was not knowledgeable, had no knowledge of the gongfu aspect of Taiji, or held back their knowledge except the teaching of the basic forms. Some didn't fully explain what they were willing to share with their students. Some Teachers only knew the basic form and got upset when someone asked a question. I was unwilling to quit and realized that in order to correct the problem I must find the right teacher(s), and travel to the epicenter of Taiji in order to see what was missing and how practitioners were trained in China.

Traveling to China renewed my faith that the art was alive and real and that the practitioners were receiving the proper training and information. I then sought out teachers who could educate me and extend my knowledge to a deeper level. This was somewhat successful since many teachers and masters in China were willing to share their knowledge with those who are sincere to learn and want to master the art. I was happy as I went to China and Hong Kong to study but I could only stay for short periods of time. I continue to go when I have a chance to where Taiji and martial arts is taken seriously amongst the students and practitioners. I also realized that all the secrecy that was there would not stop me because the real masters and teachers are willing to share and want to see students who could represent the art on a high level.

Fortunately, I have met many masters and teachers who exemplify the high art of internal martial arts and external wushu. I also realized that I must do more research and study so I could garner what I needed to know and understand. I realized this is not the most ideal way but it could help me learn what I needed in order to grow. I realized the best way was either move to China or to study and research the classics. No one mentioned that. This no way removed the need for adequate teachers of the art but was supplemental to my training. For those who do not have Teachers study the classics.

For those practitioners in the US it isn't so easy to find qualified teachers close to where you live. Even though Chinese martial arts are growing, it is being dissected as westerners dissect what should be shared as is. Instead we should be assisting in creating a community so that the growth of the art will grow and remain healthy. Westerners need to not put on its biases like it does most everything else. But I have seen it rear its ugly head. Like Wushu the right and proper teachers need to help the students to grow and proper information disseminated so everyone can excel thereby pushing the art upward and forward.

Many say that the art of Taiji in the US is weak and not very useful except as a health exercise and for competitions, which many are learning from DVD's. This is counterproductive to the art, and those masters who hold the art high in their hearts. This is also disheartening for those practitioners who practice the art for art's sake and are seeking to excel and promote the Chinese treasure. But those of us who really love the art aren't despairing since we are going to great lengths to learn, study, research, travel and help each other to grow and develop. There are a few teachers and masters who also are teaching to prove that this Chinese treasure called internal martial arts like Wushu is real and viable. It is important that the practitioners also help in order to show the high art of Taiji and serve to foster growth and sharing of the art with the rest of the world. I was fortunate that in my search and travel I was able to witness the high art lovers of Taiji and internal martial arts experts. In China and Hong Kong I witnessed the brother and sisterhood between its practitioners like one big family. I had to learn what was missing in my attempt to grow in order to become an art lover too. The need for teachers and masters willing to share all that is necessary to prove that Taiji is a high art is imperative and required. For several years I taught Taiji and tried to impart the highest standards of traditional and modern styles. I also tried to impart the principles that I learned and the WuDe (integrity and virtue.) I continue to grow and promote the high standards of teaching and sharing.

So writing this book is an attempt to foster more teachers and masters, to share vital information with its practitioners and lovers of the art. Also this book brings some important classic information together to assist all the practitioners who don't have a Teacher teaching and explaining the essential points of Taiji that are required, needed and absorbed in order to reach a high level of expertise in the practice of Taiji.

This is for art's sake and to show that Chinese treasure is a diamond and a pearl, not just a rock or unpolished stone. Not everyone wants to shine but there are those who want to just practice for health, those who want to practice to just win medals in tournaments, those who want to show the art is really a martial art capable of use as a self defense art, and then there are those who want to show that Taiji is a high art. All of these options should be realized by its practitioners and can be accomplished if we can find the vital information and the proper teachers to assist us who love to practice this art. So read these pages within and know what is required, is within these pages except a live teacher, that you must find on your own. Good journey to all and may all your dreams be realized!

A Few Insightful Observations

Those insights I have observed and learned are as follows:

- The need for qualified teachers who are willing to share their knowledge and willing to teach you so you can reach a high level.
- One must do research and continually read and understand the classic materials left by ancestors who documented what and how to do and when.
- Test oneself at different points and places in your practice so you are clear. If you have progressed and still don't understand key points outlined in the classics whether your teacher is teaching them or not.
- It is vital to use the internal martial arts to improve your health and if it is not happening, you need to see what is missing in your practice.
- If you don't understand some aspect ask someone that does, too many practitioners spend years not understanding or asking the questions they need answered. If you don't ask how you expect to gain the answer, but I do get it, one must find the one who can properly answer the question.
- Harmony within is important because nature requires harmony and so do we.
- Understand the heart and the spiritual within your practice especially as you progress to higher levels.
- Movement is in stillness and in stillness there is movement. One part moves and all parts move (一动全动).

Further Insight

There is much to learn, and even more to be absorbed so it is important to study, and research unless you are not that interested or you are fortunate to have a teacher who has explained everything to you. Most masters in Chinese martial arts or Wushu expect one to study even as they learn and practice with their Master teacher. I have found that if you feel something is missing in your practice or you are not growing you must study the classics to fill that void. Study of the classics will give you insight into what may be lacking. If not you can ask your teacher who may impart the necessary knowledge. The other point is that even if you study, you have to figure out how to incorporate those ingredients into your practice and master them. The easy way is to be guided by a Teacher. The other is to practice until you are able to exhibit what you have learned. One of the things I also found that was a great help, is to go over the classics not only once, but many times in order to be clear, and understand Taijiquan.

Taiji uses "emptiness and stillness" as its main principle. Every movement focuses on softness and dismissive of hardness. Those who fall in love with the external posture don't understand Taijiquan, for the supreme achievement of this art is the cultivation of spirit. Taijiquan emphasizes the cultivation of both body and mind. The classics state, when practicing, you must "use mind to move the energy, and use energy to move your body." The classics say, consciousness and energy are the rulers, the mind is the commander; energy is the signal banner; bones and muscles, are the administrators. This philosophy identifies Taijiquan as a total martial arts system that includes the body, mind, energy and consciousness as all working together as one in unison.

Its fighting method is not a matter of winning through strength, but by skills and techniques. You now adequately know the special characteristics of this art. All martial and boxing arts have their merits, their strengths and weaknesses, their focuses, and their special characteristics. Taijiquan is no different. Taiji has its martial arts and healing abilities that can be developed simultaneously.

Chopsticks

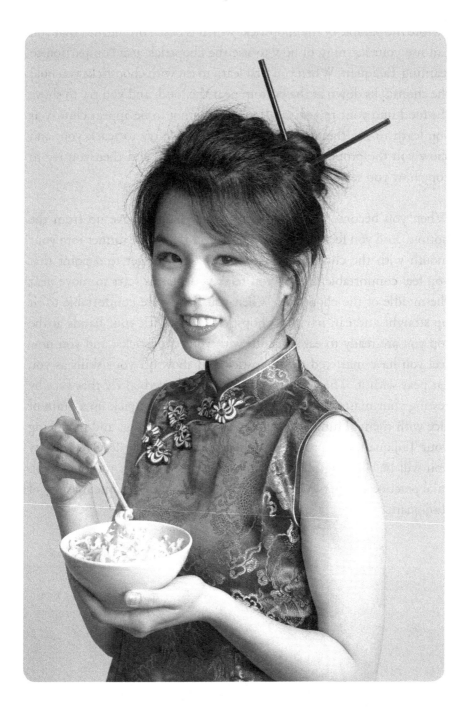

Conclusion: The Parable of the Chopstick

I wrote the parable of the chopstick, which is based on the idea that you can use your learning of how to use the chopstick as a comparison to learning Taijiquan. When you first learn to eat with chopsticks you hold the chopsticks down at the bottom near the food, and you try to shove the food into your mouth while you trying not to be appear clumsy as you learn to use the chopstick properly. People try to teach you, and show you the proper technique as you continue, and then you try to copy how you see others using the chopsticks.

When you become a little proficient your hands move up from the bottom, and you feel confident you can get the whole dinner into your mouth with the chopsticks. As you practice you get to a point that you feel comfortable, and as you relax your hands start to move near the middle of the chopstick. When you finally are comfortable to sit up straight and can navigate chopsticks easily with your hands at the top you are ready to eat soft tofu with your chopsticks, and you now feel you have mastered the chopstick and show off your skills as you eat peas with it. Then you try to catch the proverbial fly that flies by testing your mastery of the chopstick until you can pick up a grain of rice with them. Think about it when you are learning, and practicing your Taijiquan, and progressing through the different levels. One day you will be showing off your chopstick mastery skills too but it will take practice and perseverance. The same is required in the mastery of Taijiquan.

II

THE PRACTICE
Lian Xi

The Practice

The practice of Taijiquan starts with proper training, which cannot be skipped. Training is required even at the mastery level just like any other form of exercise. It is ideal to practice everyday, doing something such as Zhanzhuang, or silk reeling or forms, weapons, refining your form, applications or fundamentals that you have learned from your teacher. Since Taijiquan requires a deep understanding, and requires consistent practice you must commit to the long haul as opposed to only short term training then thinking you know it all or that all you need to learn is the form and it is sufficient to master Taijiquan.

Practice does make perfect, and if you practice you will see your movement toward perfection. There are many levels of practice and perfection, which we will discuss later but suffice to say you must practice, and continue to grow through practice. In internal martial arts there is much to learn, and it requires a lot of practice to perfect your art. What to practice is equally important as what to train, on any given day. It is important to practice and is vital in order to reach a level of mastery or art. The big question comes down to what to train, and when so that you can progress steadily upward toward the goals you are trying to reach. There are different criteria for mastery, or competition, or self-defense, or good health to name a few.

The Training

Training to become a master in internal arts or Taijiquan we must start at the beginning even though when reading this book you may have already started your training or deep into your practice. So don't be concerned if we cover some material you are familiar with because there may be material new to you or reinforces what you already know. So let's begin, training by teachers may differ but eventually, they may cover the same material or types of training. It depends on your teachers' goal, experience and/or focus. For example, if your teacher focuses on training you to compete in competitions then they may focus on the forms training, and their only concern is that you learn the form, and the structure of the forms, and how it will look when you compete to win gold metal. That type of teacher focuses on the perfection of what the forms looks like, and the structure of it. You may have a teacher who focuses on health preservation, and doesn't care about what the perfection of the forms looks like. They are only focused on the exercise as it pertains to health. Other teachers who are martial artists, and want to teach you the martial aspects will focus on the forms but add the requirements of the self-defense aspects, which may include some fighting techniques. Each of these teachers will teach you what is their focus or purpose for teaching their students Taijiquan. Your first requirement should be to understand what your teacher's focus or purpose is. If your teacher wants to train a student to become a master then the training will be more comprehensive, and take a level of dedication from you, and a variety of lessons over a long period of time. This will require your commitment to train, learn, and practice for a very long time. Some teachers will teach you according to your ability, commitment, your heart, and proof that you will hang in there for the long haul, and you will practice diligently so as to not waste their time, and energy.

The second important thing is to understand when you are training in internal arts it requires you to learn, and understand there are different levels of training, and must not think like some that soon as you learn a form, think that you are at the master level or you are a master because you won a medal at a competition.

The first level of basic training normally will be to require you to stretch, and loosen up, practice some preliminary or single basic forms. If you have never practiced a martial art form of any kind I suggest you start at the very basic level, and then practice, and progress slowly. The beginning of any martial art is to begin with basic training to prepare your foundation. Foundation training is best because you then are at the place to start to prepare your body and mind, the same as building a house you must start at the foundation. Once completing the foundation exercises you can progress to the next level of learning forms depending on the form(s) you are now committed to learn. For senior citizens it is important to stretch, practice slow and pay attention to your body so it can tell you what is happening. The slow practice will help remove any blockages and old baggage, which can get in the way of the smooth flow of Qi energy. It will also help identify where there are old injuries and debris left behind that need to be removed. This takes time and the slow practice and foundational exercises will help to clear the way for your circulation to improve thereby improving your overall health.

What are Foundational Exercises?

Foundational exercises are the type of exercises that you practice to limber up, stretch, and learn how to stand, how to move, your body, feet, hands, and any basic requirements to practice that particular art form you are learning. At the same time internal martial arts will require you to stand and practice Zhanzhuang (standing pole) training in order to begin to understand that internal requirements, a strong foundation, rooting, relaxation, and how to begin to build your energy. Many teachers, who don't realize this is vital to internal gongfu practice, sometimes skip this step. If this is left out you may be missing a vital ingredient that will be felt later on in your practice. Since we are discussing the art, and mastery then it is required for the practitioner to practice the art of Zhanzhuang. If you are only for competition then some teachers don't require it, but I will disagree, and say it is required for all practitioners of any internal gongfu practice.

When you are training, be clear about what you are studying, and what level you are at. Don't try and rush past or skip the basic foundation training. The reason for this is that many practitioners practice but never progress to higher levels because they are always training at the same one level, and don't realize it until years later, and blame their teacher for it having never asked or enquired about reaching any other level.

Learning the Basics

The basics; start with foundation exercises, and then forms training to begin to learn different movements step by step. Once a basic form is being learned one should endeavor to perform it properly, and practice each new form or movement until it is ingrained into you. They say practice a new form everyday for 100 days, and you will remember it, 1000 days, and you won't forget it, it is your form now. Be not fooled if you want to own the forms, then you have to train and practice everyday for the rest of your life so consider what you are learning is now your daily/weekly practice. With internal martial arts the more you practice the more you will continue to grow. Also paying attention to the Classics will assist you in your mastery of Taijiquan so we must start with incorporating essential lessons from the Masters.

Types of Forms to Learn

There are several major Taiji forms such as Chen, Wu, Wu (Hao), Sun, Yang and Wudang styles. Each offer different ways to practice but the essential basic foundation are the same no matter which forms you choose to practice. The emphasis is different in each style because the premise to create a new form was to focus on a different aspect coupled with previous training of the master who created it. The principles are the same but Masters sometimes create new styles in order to focus on their goals or knowledge they are trying to impart. Remember first there was one now there are several styles but the principles remain the same.

Which is the Best Form?

The best form(s) is the form(s) you choose to learn, because they are all based upon a similar foundation and set of principles. Choose the one(s) that you prefer or try out different ones until you decide which one you like. Like a car we all like different vehicles, makes and models but all of them will get us to our destination.

Why Train and Practice Forms

The forms practice is a set of instructional postures that will guide you to learning the internal martial art of Taijiquan. The forms will effectively lead you to learn and understand, the movements, the uses and how to utilize each posture in the forms. The postures are strung together but can be practiced alone as each one is an entire posture and practice unto itself. The postures are strung together the same way you will string along beads of a necklace or chain. One posture leads to another and should be practiced like that seamlessly until smooth till the end. Then one should practice each posture internally the same way as if one is stringing each joint together as if all the joints are connected like a string of pearls. One should try to perfect the different postures. Understanding the meaning of the posture and why it was given its' name and how it is accomplished within the 13 energies will be helpful.

The Form: What to Gain and What to Lose

What is gained is the ability to learn a martial art and how one can learn to flow smoothly transitioning from one form or movement to the next like a silk reeling worm. When practicing the forms one will gain knowledge, and experience, learning how to utilize the skills of the martial art of Taijiquan. What is lost if you don't learn how to practice each form correctly? It may lead you away from your goal of learning how to use the postures and how to master the techniques of the forms when you are required to apply them.

Insight

Along with learning the postures completely it is good to learn the applications. Also we must be able to practice in a way that the flow of energy is smooth and unbroken within the body and the mind (yi意) and everything is connected together like the links in a chain or a string of pearls. We want to gain a good practice and we want to eliminate any faults or bad practices such as listed in the ten essential points, and the practice of the thirteen postures. Practice slowly until one understands how to accomplish and be mindful of the posture, your internal system and the essential points.

Type of Frames in Taijiquan

Most people won't discuss the types of Taiji when it comes to the type of circle (frame) you learn and/or practice. We can talk about the styles of Taiji such as Wu or Yang style but one should understand the type of circle also. Why you say? Most Teachers and students don't choose the type of training they seek within the style because we learn and practice whatever style our Teacher knows or is willing to teach us. Teachers typically teach whatever style they either know or what they think the student can learn and master given the student's skill level or competency. There is big frame (circle), middle frame and small frame. There is a distinct difference between the three frames and normally the big frame is considered to be for health or for beginners and the middle frame is considered for those students that are at the intermediate level and small frame is considered to be for more advanced practitioners and for gaining more self defense or combat skills. I think all three require the same principles but the difference between making large circles or small circles is one of learning and skill levels. Some Teachers who only know the small frame forms will only teach those and some big frame Teachers only teach big frame forms. Some styles lean toward big frame such as Chen style basic forms such as Laojia and Yang style forms whereas styles such as Wu style and Zhaobao are small frames. Chen and Yang also have large, middle and small frames. A master in Chen Village explained to me that if one learned how to make a big circle then one can learn to make small circles but if one learns small circles one will not make big circles. When one thinks about it makes perfect sense so it may be best to learn large frame (circle) first then progress to small frame (circle).

Some Masters say it is a matter of progression in your training so if you start with large circle these will eventually become small circles. Others say small frame is more for combat but if one understands the principles then all boats will eventually reach the same port. Also it should be mentioned that there are slow forms and fast forms. Many practitioners only learn or know the slow forms but one should endeavor to learn and practice the fast forms because they help the practitioners to improve their speed, endurance and power such as Paochui. It doesn't mean you cannot practice the slow forms fast. I recommend you do both slow and fast but one must preserve the integrity of the principles slow or fast. You can discuss with your Teacher the styles, the frames and the slow and fast forms but it is important to know of their existence. So let's understand the principles, as written, in the classics.

Wudan Style Taiji (Jian)

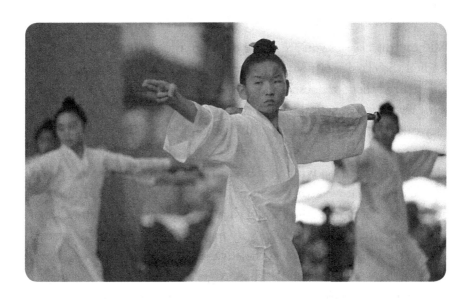

Understanding The Classics

If you want to learn to master Taijiquan or any internal martial art one must study the classics for they represent the innate wisdom teachings left behind for all students to be able to understand and progress to become proficient in the art. Understanding the wisdom of the classics, earlier teachers and masters created a body of information, and instructions that explain the foundation of Taijiquan and its important points that one should know. The rest can be imparted to you via a teacher, and your own research.

Without the classics you are at the mercy of the teacher who may have studied the classics or not, and after studying them still haven't either internalized them or doesn't know them at all. This has happened since some teachers focus on the modern aspects of Taiji, and focus on what they call the performance art solely for competition or those who only do the form as a way of basic physical exercise. If Taiji is just a physical exercise form then studying the classics is not a priority for some. Many people think that what they see is what they get but the intrinsic values of Taiji, is hidden from the view of the eyes because many cannot see or understand the invisible. Hence why many say the real Taiji is encased in secrecy. This may be true at the advanced levels but the classics help to share the vital and essential knowledge. If you are seeking to master Taijiquan or expect to become a Taiji Master of the art then you must research, and understand the classics otherwise you are leaving the brick with no mortar. Listed below is some valuable information that you need to read and learn or review as a Taiji practitioner, teacher or artist.

What is the most important reason of the Classics? Show you the way, the path and make the journey fruitful so that you will receive the basics (foundation) needed to practice the high art of Taiji. Also the classics will help one to correct major mistakes and clear up some confusion. Be careful though the classics, is what the masters learned, experienced and observed. So some of these classics have to be interpreted properly in order to fully understand what the ancient Masters are trying to share. The idea that there is a string pulling you up is about Qi pulling you up and the need to insure you keep your head up and chin in but not by force, it is done naturally. So do not deform your body such as when one forcibly tucks in their butt, or squeeze your toes, or sinking the chest and rounding the back. It should all be done in a relaxed natural mode. Actually you are not supposed to stress or put tension on your body. Your teacher will do the rest. The first order of business is to learn and understand these treatises:

Taijiquan Jing

(Attributed to Chang San-feng (est. 1279 -1386) as researched by Lee N. Scheele)

In motion the whole body should be light and agile, with all parts of the body linked as if threaded together.

The *Qi* [vital life energy] should be excited, The *shen* (spirit of vitality) should be internally gathered.

The postures should be without defect, without hollows or projections from the proper alignment; in motion the Form should be continuous, without stops and starts.

The *Jin* (intrinsic strength) should be rooted in the feet, generated from the legs, controlled by the waist, and manifested through the fingers.

The feet, legs, and waist should act together as an integrated whole, so that while advancing or withdrawing one can grasp the opportunity of favorable timing and advantageous position.

If correct timing and position are not achieved, the body will become disordered and will not move as an integrated whole; the correction for this defect must be sought in the legs and waist.

The principle of adjusting the legs and waist applies for moving in all directions; upward or downward, advancing or withdrawing, left or right.

All movements are motivated by I (Yi) (mind-intention,) not external form.

If there is up, there is down; when advancing have regard for withdrawing; when striking left, pay attention to the right.

If the I (Yi), wants to move upward, it must simultaneously have intent downward.

Alternating the force of pulling and pushing severs an opponent's root so that he can be defeated quickly and certainly.

Insubstantial and substantial should be clearly differentiated. At any place where there is insubstantiality, there must be substantiality; Every place has both insubstantiality and substantiality.

The whole body should be threaded together through every joint without the slightest break.

Chang quan [Long Boxing] is like a great river rolling on unceasingly.

Peng, Lu, Qi, An, Ts'ai, Lie, Zhou, and *K'ao* are equated to the Eight Trigrams. The first four are the cardinal directions; *Qian* [South; Heaven], *K'un* [North; Earth], *K'an* [West; Water], and *Li* [East; Fire]. The second four are the four corners: *Sun* [Southwest; Wind], *Chen* [Northeast; Thunder], *Tui* [Southeast; Lake], and *Ken* [Northwest; Mountain]. Advance (*Jin*), Withdraw (*T'ui*), Look Left (*Tso Ku*), Look Right (*Yu Pan*), and Central Equilibrium (*Chung Ting*) are equated to the five elements: Metal, Wood, Water, Fire, and Earth All together these are termed the Thirteen Postures

(A footnote appended to this Classic by Yang Lu-chan (1799-1872) reads: This treatise was left by the patriarch Chan San feng of Wu Tang Mountain, with a desire toward helping able people everywhere to have longevity, and not merely as a means to martial skill.)

Insight

In the Taijiquan Jing one must endeavor to read and test to insure you can meet these essential keys and not assume you are doing everything it says. This treatise is trying to insure you are sinking mentally and you are light on top, heavy on the bottom. It is also trying to insure when you practice the postures you are moving correctly and are paying attention to such things as yin, yang; substantial and insubstantial. If not it will show up in your applications or in your push hands practice as a defect. So study and make sure you are adhering to the key points of this classic treatise. From this one must insure the postures of the form are being done correctly by studying the classic *The Ten Essentials of Taijiquan.*

Grandmaster Yang Chengfu

Yang-single (restoration)Public Domain

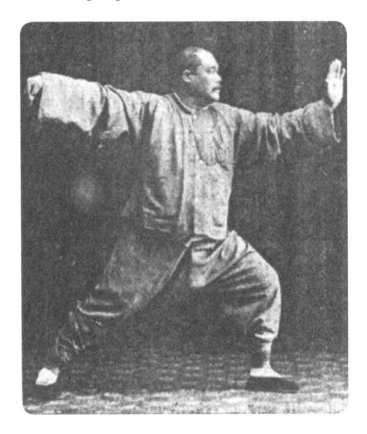

The Ten Essentials of Taijiquan Theory

(Dictated by Yang Chengfu, recorded by Chen Weiming)

1. ***An intangible and lively energy lifts the crown of the head.*** This refers to holding the head in vertical alignment, with the spirit threaded to the top of the head. One must not use strength; using strength will stiffen the neck and inhibit the flow of Qi and blood. One must have the conscious intent of an intangible, lively, and natural phenomenon. If not, then the vital energy (jingshen) will not be able to rise.

2. ***Contain the chest and raise the back.*** "Containing the chest" means hold in the chest slightly to allow the Qi to sink to dantian. One must avoid rigidity in the chest; thrusting out the chest will cause blockage in the chest cavity. One will be heavy above and light below; the heels will float up. "Raise the back" means the Qi adheres to the back. If one is able to contain the chest, then one will naturally be able to raise the back. If one can raise the back, the strength will be able to issue from the spine, and you will be undefeatable.

3. ***Relax the waist.*** The waist is the body's ruler. If you are able to relax the waist, the two feet will have strength and the foundation will be stable. The changes of insubstantial and substantial all come from turning the waist, hence it is said, "The source of meaning is in the region of one's waist." If there is a situation in which you are unable to attain strength, you must seek the cause in the waist.

4. ***Distinguish insubstantial and substantial.*** The art of Taijiquan takes the distinction between insubstantial and substantial as the first principle. If the weight of the entire body is placed over the right leg, then the right leg is substantial and the left is empty. If the entire body's weight is placed over the left leg, then the left leg

is substantial and the right leg is empty. If one is able to distinguish empty and full, the body's turning motions will be light and agile, and there will be no wasted strength. If one is unable to distinguish, one's step will be heavy and sluggish, one's stance will be unsteady, and one will easily be unbalanced by an opponent's pull.

5. ***Sink the shoulders and drop the elbows.*** "Sink the shoulders" means the shoulders are relaxed, open, and allowed to hang down. If one is unable to relax and allow the two shoulders to hang down, they will rise up, then the Qi will also follow them up, and the whole body will lack strength. "Dropping the elbows," means relaxing the elbows downward, and letting the hang. If the elbows are drawn up, then the shoulders will be unable to sink, and you will not be able to push an opponent far. Isn't this similar to the short energy of the external martial arts?

6. ***Use consciousness, not strength.*** This is spoken of in the "Taijiquan Classics." This is entirely the use of mind/intent (yi), not use of strength (li). In practicing *Taijiquan*, the entire body is loosened (song) and open; avoid the use of the slightest bit of crude force (zhuo li), which causes blockage in the sinews, bones and blood vessels, and causes one to be bound up. Then you will enable a light agility in the changes, and the circular rotations will come freely. Some doubt: without using strength, how can one increase one's strength? Now, the human body has meridians – as with the Earth's watercourses, when the watercourses are unblocked, the water flows. When the meridians are unblocked, then the Qi passes through. If the whole body is stiff, the *Jin* fills the meridians, the Qi and blood become stagnant, and the turning motions are not nimble. If one hair is pulled, the whole body is moved. If one does not use strength but instead use mind/intent (yi), then where the yi arrives, the Qi follows. If the Qi and the blood flow fully, daily threading and flowing through the entire body, there will be no time when there are blockages. After a long practice, one then

attains genuine internal strength. Hence, the statement in the "Taijiquan Classics": "Arriving at the extreme of yielding softness, one afterward arrives at the extreme of solid hardness." The arms of those who are proficient in the skill of *Taijiquan* are like iron within cotton, and extremely heavy. When practitioners of external martial arts use strength, then their strength is evident. When not using strength, they are light and floating. It is obvious that their strength remains an outward energy, as surface energy. When not using mind/intent (yi) but using strength, it is very easy to be led in – this is not worthy of respect.

7. ***Upper and lower follow one another.*** Upper and lower follow one another is what is referred to in the saying from the "Taijiquan Classics"; It is rooted in the feet, issued by the legs, governed by the waist, expressed in the fingers. From the feet, to the legs, then to the waist, always there must be complete integration into one Qi." With the movements of the hands, waist, and feet, the focus of the eyes, also follow their movements. When it is like this, only then can it be called "upper and lower follow each other." If there is one part that does not move, then the form is scattered and confused.

8. ***Internal and external are united.*** What one trains in *Taijiquan* is the spirit, therefore it is said, "The spirit isn't the leader, and the body follows its order." If one is able to raise the spirit of vitality, one will naturally be able to deport oneself lightly and with agility. The form is none other than empty, full, open and closed. What is called open is not only the opening of the hands and the feet – the mind/intent also opens with them accordingly. What is called closing of the hands and feet – the mind/intent also closes with them accordingly. When able to unite inner with outer as one Qi, then there is complete continuity.

9. ***Linked without breaks.*** With practitioners of external martial arts, their strength is contrived and crude force (hou tian zhi zhuo

li). Therefore it has it starts and stops, its duration and cessation. When it's old strength is already depleted, its new strength has not yet been born. At these times it is most easily overcome. Taijiquan uses mind/intent, not strength. From beginning to finish it is continuous without ceasing, a complete cycle back to the beginning, circling without end. In the original teachings it is said: "Like the Long River, it flows smoothly on without ceasing." It is also said, "Move the jin [energy] as though drawing silk [from a cocoon]." These words refer to its being threaded together (guan chuan) as one Qi.

10. **Seek stillness in motion.** The External martial arts view leaping and tumbling as ability. They employ exertion of Qi and strength, so that after training they are invariably gasping for breath. *Taijiquan* uses stillness to manage movement. Even when there is movement there is stillness. Therefore, in practicing the form, the slower the better. When practicing slowly, the breathing deepens and lengthens, the Qi sinks to the dantian. One avoids the harm of straining the blood circulation. Students should carefully contemplate this, so as to attain it's meaning.

(Reference: Master Yang Style Taijiquan by Fu Zhongwen translated by Louis Swaim ISBN 9781583941522)

Insight

Is the crown of your head being lifted by the intrinsic energy rising to the top? Is your waist relaxed? These ten essential points will help you to identify what you are doing correctly or not in the practice of the postures. One must learn and study the Classics judiciously and not skimp on this because the Classics direct our understanding of the internal art forms of Taiji. Something as simple as there is stillness in motion and visa versa should be contemplated and made sure we can fully agree with that point. Just like there should be no breaks, check yourself to see if you comply with this point when practicing your forms.

Read and digest the classics as if you are trying to master the best dish your family cooks in order to prove you have learned its methods and can duplicate their cooking or exceed it. Many times we taste great dishes at the restaurant but when we try it at home it doesn't taste the same. We buy the cookbook but still can't duplicate the taste of the dish we are preparing so we have to continually try and study to see what ingredient was left out (hence the secret ingredient) until we can discover it and learn what is missing. (Truth is, they always leave out one ingredient on purpose). Once we learn what is missing we can then add the essential ingredients, and make the perfect dish. The same in Taiji, we must study the classics and garner all we can from them until we can perfect our practice of Taiji. At the same time we must be aware of the three fears and the three faults and try to eliminate the three faults.

The Three Fears

Master Cheng talks about not fearing anything….

1. One must not fear bitter work: hard work is bitter
2. One should not fear losing: one must lose to gain
3. One should not fear ferocity: stay relaxed no matter who comes to attack

The Three Faults

*Master Cheng talks about eliminating three faults before you can learn Taiji. It goes something like this. You **MUST** overcome three cardinal faults to become successful at cultivating Taiji.*

1: "The first fault is lack of perseverance".

I think I can sum it up like this:
When you learn a new posture: PRACTICE
When you forget a new posture: PRACTICE
When you think you remember a new posture: PRACTICE
When you think you have it right: PRACTICE
When you are sure you don't have it right: PRACTICE
When you feel good about your Taiji: PRACTICE
When you are bored with your Taiji: PRACTICE
When you are happy with your Taiji: PRACTICE
When you are frustrated: PRACTICE
When there is no class on any given day: PRACTICE
When you get up in the morning: PRACTICE
When you want to go to sleep at night, take a bit of time and: PRACTICE
When you are feeling refreshed: PRACTICE
When you are tired: PRACTICE
When you have an excuse not to: PRACTICE

2. "The second fault is greed"

Do not bite off more than you can chew.

If you were taught three postures and can only remember one, practice what you can remember and wing it the rest of the way. You can be assured the instructor will correct you next time you see him/her. That's why they are called instructors.

Don't jump ahead faster than you can absorb. I don't care if it takes all summer to learn the Grasp Sparrow's Tail Sequence. If you can do it better than anybody I know, you are a step ahead. Take baby steps. A little bit well, is way better than a lot done poorly, and you will be better for it.

When you are learning a sequence, take one posture at a time and practice it until you feel it. Then take a second posture and do the same. Then take both of them and glue them together with whatever feels right. Correct that and start again with another move. Enjoy yourself. Making mistakes can be fun and you will find that there are multiple ways to get to your desired result. If you are too greedy, and bite off more than you can digest, you are guaranteed indigestion. You will frustrate yourself and quit. All this is because you were too greedy. Take your time. Learn it well, and right, even if it is more slowly. Enjoy yourself. Chill baby!

3. "The third fault is impatience"

Don't be in a rush. You are far better to take a couple of years to learn a form than to learn it badly. That is one of the problems with big classes. They make you feel like an idiot if you don't keep up. Everyone has difficulty with something. When I was learning, I had a terrible time with the Fair Lady sequence. I couldn't make it flow. One weekend I found myself with free time so I locked myself in to my little basement with a couple of DVD's. I watched and copied at first. Then I put the DVD's away and tried by myself. I was terrible. I could not make it flow. I tried an experiment. First I made sure my footwork was right. Once I had that down, I put a couple of tunes on my IPod. Suddenly it flowed. Wow. Then I tried it without music. It still flowed. It's now one of my favorite parts of the form. So, don't be impatient. Just keep practicing. Think out of the box. Ask a buddy to help you. Whatever it takes.

(Master Cheng also had one other important tip. He recognized that we are not all necessarily gifted in the same way. He said, "If it is your fate to be a little dull, just work ten times harder than anyone else." Take my word for it, he is right.)

Insight

It does not matter how long it takes to learn something. Once you have learned it, it is the same as anyone else. As a practitioner do not fear any hard work or anyone. Always remain calm in the face of adversity. As a teacher, I do not give a hoot how long you take to learn something. It is the student that becomes aware of these faults and has eliminated them that will succeed. We don't want to have any faults that will steer us in the wrong direction or keep us from improving and growing in our practice. Additional insight and important instructions are revealed via the classics and they try to explain what some teachers try to teach their students or knowledge that some teachers do not impart. It is important to do your own research and study to complement your training including any faults to be aware as listed above. Below is additional classical knowledge of the *Thirteen Postures* for one to study and ponder.

Master Siu Fong Evans

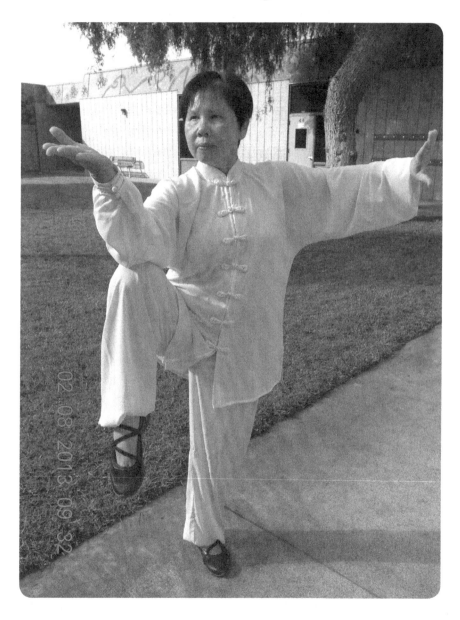

Song of The Thirteen Postures

十三總勢莫輕視，命意源頭在腰隙。

變轉虛實須留意，氣遍身軀不稍癡。

靜中觸動動猶靜，因敵變化是神奇。

勢勢存心揆用意，得來不覺費工夫。

刻刻留心在腰間，腹內鬆淨氣騰然。

尾閭中正神貫頂，滿身輕利頂頭懸。

仔細留心向推求，屈伸開合聽自由。

入門引路須口授，工用無息法自休。

若言體用何為準，意氣君來骨肉臣。

詳推用意終何在，益壽延年不老春。

歌兮歌兮百四十，字字真切義無遺。

若不向此推求去，枉費功夫遺嘆息。

Song of The Thirteen Postures

(by Unknown Author as researched by Lee N. Scheele English translation)

The Thirteen Postures should not be taken lightly; the source of the postures is in the waist.

Be mindful of the interchange between insubstantial and substantial; the Qi circulates throughout the body without hindrance.

Be still, when attacked by the opponent, be tranquil and move in stillness; changes caused by my opponent fill him with wonder.

Study the function of each posture carefully and with deliberation; to achieve the goal is very easy.

Pay attention to the waist at all times; completely relax the abdomen and the Qi rises up.

When the tailbone is centered and straight, the shen (spirit of vitality) goes through to the head top.

To make the whole body light and agile suspend the head top.

Carefully study, extension and contraction, opening and closing, should be natural.

To enter the door and be shown the way, you must be orally taught. Practice should be uninterrupted, and technique achieved by self-study.

Speaking of the body and its function, what is the standard?

The I (yi-mind-intent) and Qi are king, and the bones and muscles are the court.

Think over carefully what the final purpose is: to lengthen life and maintain youth.

The Song consists of 140 characters; each character is true and the meaning is complete.

If you do not study in this manner, then you will waste your time and sigh with regret.

Insight

The classics are available in order to assist all Taiji practitioners with the required knowledge in order to grow with or without a qualified teacher. Some practitioners, have a qualified teacher, some have none. Both should still read and research the classics, which will provide valuable knowledge in order to help practitioners on their path toward mastery. Go over the classics until you can internalize them within your practice. What you skip over might be the answer you are seeking. If you find parts of the classics you don't understand or currently not doing determine how to add to your training. Later on we will discuss a deeper explanation of the thirteen postures in the Classic: *Expositions of Insights into the Practice of the Thirteen Postures,* which focuses on the internal practice.

Tasting the Bitter Before the Sweet

Once when talking with Master Chen Xiaoxing (Headmaster at Chen Village), I questioned the training and the growth and mastery ability of western Taiji practitioners. He stated that the basic difference was something called "tasting the bitter before the sweet." I enquired as to what was the meaning of this. Master Chen explained that the training in China required a lot of tough training, extensive practice because the local practitioners spend a majority of their time training with the Master Teachers. They also practice on their own for countless hours and corrections until they can do it correctly. Aside from that when not learning or practicing their art of Chen style Taiji the students and families have to work in the fields growing and harvesting food and vegetables. Also, the Taiji practitioners have a lot of tough competition to compete and compare to. For example if you live in a community where everyone have practiced Taiji for generations you can't take learning the art of your ancestors, and elders lightly. This is considered a national treasure and it is not practiced only as a sport. In the West many people practice lightly because of their multi faceted lifestyle and they do not have to prove they are the next lineage holder for the community or province. In the west you have to try to do the same even if you do not realize it, especially if you practice by yourself or with a Teacher who is not a high level master. So you must persevere and patiently practice.

Insight

Now understand the real meaning of bitter also expresses the level of practice and patience one must experience on the road to mastering the art of Taijiquan. If you do not live in China or do not have a High-level Master Teacher, or you practice by yourself, you should still practice, research and continue practicing until you realize your goals. When doing this you are "tasting some of the bitter." When you try to understand the classics and internalize them in your practice you are fulfilling the requirements necessary to advance, and increase your abilities. It takes time, practice, and patience in order to master Taiji. The training and continued practice and patience is the bitter. As you gain knowledge and practice the art, that is, tasting the sweet. Some may think the sweet is the training, and then participating in a competition. Winning medals is the sweet, and it is, but if you have only medals but have not mastered the art, then enjoy the sweet success. Ask where is the bitter at the next level.

Additional Foundational Training

Additional training is required in order to master Taijiquan so review the following list to insure it is included in your practice or identify what you need to add:

Zhanzhuang (Standing Pole (Post) Training

Standing stake or pole is an essential exercise that is utilized to help improve a persons' ability to relax, develop a root, increase circulation and increase the development of Qi. Also Santi stance is similar and beneficial to help one sink their Qi and gain more internal strength. Should you do standing post or not is up to you and/or your Teacher.

Stretching

Stretching is advisable essential exercises in order to help stretch and protect the muscles, ligaments, tendons and joints. Start slowly and do not over stretch. Later on you can learn to do power stretching.

Meditation

Basic meditation is used to help relax a person, increase Qi, calm the mind, focus the mind-intent, and help basic circulation. There are also many meditative exercises that help heal practitioners.

Basic Wushu and foundation training

Basic Wushu exercises are vital as a basis for practicing martial arts. You can't convince me you are a martial artist if you can't make a proper fist.

Basic Qigong training

Basic energy training helps to heal and increase the vital Qi of practitioners, vital for the practice of Taiji.

Correction

Correction is vital as practitioners train in order to insure that form postures and movements are completed correctly. Corrections are important because it will improve Qi flow and help with the applications that otherwise may have failed.

Unitized Movement

When one part moves does all parts move? If not then practice more. When one part stops does the other parts stop? If not practice more. All parts of the body should move together as one.

Testing

Testing includes demonstration of the postures, movement transitions, and how techniques are utilized in Taiji. Testing is for self-evaluation in order to clear up the misconception as to your progress such as where are you really as opposed to what and where you think you are. Use testing as a tool since you must know yourself. Practitioners should assist in the testing of each other.

What to Test

Testing is imperative for those practitioners who want to master Taiji. This is why practitioners must give up their ego for success and test each other, which will help you to grow. If you are only practicing for health then it is not vital to test. If you are seeking to master the art or use it for self-defense then it behooves you to test when you can. Testing requires you test as follows and much more:

- ✓ Stance for rooting -front, back, side, up, down
- ✓ Balance for stability -two legs, one leg, arms
- ✓ Each posture moving and still
- ✓ For Li or Peng jin
- ✓ Test anyplace touch on body touch ground (advance level)
- ✓ Release of tension and ice in joints
- ✓ Test for relaxation, Song
- ✓ Test for substantial versus insubstantial

Flow Analysis (my own test)

One must remove tension and blocked qi from the three gates, in shoulder, neck, and hip. This is another requirement and test.

This is advance testing but vital to check how the Qi is flowing throughout the body to check if there are any blocks inhibiting Qi flow and keeping the practitioners' health from improving or where there is hidden ice preventing progress. This can be accomplished by many Master teachers, who can reveal the same data, to assist you in being aware of potential problems.

Weapons

Weapons training, is essential as one moves from basic into advanced training. The importance is how to use weapons training to improve ones' practice. Weapons are used as a training tool and extension of your body and mind.

Push hands (advanced training)

Push hands (tsou) is advanced training that moves a practitioner from form to function and teaches one how to utilize Taiji or any internal arts as a martial art. Also pushing hands reveal what is lacking in your forms practice.

Insight

The importance of foundational training cannot be overemphasized. Without these additional components one will be missing essential core training that is vital in order to insure you can perform all of the internal and external requirements of a Taiji practitioner. Internal martial arts requires the ability to relax, be calm, clear and focus the mind intent, develop Qi energy, circulate the Qi and blood within, clear any blockages, melt any ice, and opening of the joints. Additionally one must utilize correction and testing to insure they are performing Taiji correctly. Testing and push hands is vital in order to confirm you are practicing your forms correctly and are in keeping with the essential principles of Taijiquan. There may be other items your Teacher may add according to your level in order to assist you in your mastery of Taijiquan such as Chansijin training.

Silk Reeling

What is Silk Reeling?

If you ever saw a silk worm, the silk they produce is wound onto a spindle by unwrapping the silk from their bodies. The silk comes off in one long thread until one reaches the end. The idea of wrapping oneself in silk is tantamount to one wrapping their self in energy. This also explains how our practice of Chansijin (spiral power) or Silk Reeling helps us to develop our energy and how the energy circulates in a ball. Silk Reeling includes twining, spiraling, coiling, winding, reeling and circling methods. It is required that when you move you are moving in the way of the circle or spiral. Also we need to practice until we develop unit force whereby when we turn like the ball, and any part one touches, they will spiral out of or be thrown out. Not just the dantian spirals but also the whole body can spiral. If you want to see a silkworm visit China then you will clearly understand.

Liu Hong Cai, Chen Style, on Silk Reeling describes two types of silk reeling, one is a wrapping type of energy 'doing' the movement and the second is 'using' it to affect another. He stresses that you have to understand energy to apply silk reeling. Silk reeling is a gathering and closing of energy, or power in spiraling movement. Energy manifests itself differently in different people. Whatever form it takes (silk reeling) you must learn to maintain the feeling and gain control of it as it happens to you when you're doing the form. Circulate Qi through the body so that it passes through the body to apply. The feeling, or the energy, has to arrive at the exact point (dao wei到位) not just inside the body. The ball turns at every point as the energy spirals.

Insight

The yin yang symbol depicts a circle that spirals with no end insight. Chen style Taiji emphases this via Chansijing training but this is included in all Taiji and internal styles even if not externally evident. Chen style focuses on practicing chansijing with the practice of dantian gong training. Making the dantian move with our chanjijing is vital in order to move our energy throughout our body and the meridians. There are many levels of Chansijin so one must practice and understand that when one part moves all parts move. Also one must distinguish between moving like a snake or whether one is at a higher level and can move like a dragon. Dragon is a higher level. Also there are two types of Chansijin, one you practice by yourself and the other you can use against the opponent. First learn the first step (like a snake) then later learn the more advanced spiral jin (Dragon and tornado) training. So take the time to learn how to put chansijin into every Taiji move from dantian gong training, which is taught along with other advanced skills such as Chin Na.

Chin Na

Chin Na training is a method of defense and offense that uses the methods of Chansijin and spiral jin to lock the opponents joints or limbs. Chin Na means seize control and can be as simple as locking the wrist joint to higher skills that include using internal powers. Chin Na is applied when an opponent touches you and then by using speed and spiral jin one can lock the opponent. It does not matter where the opponent touches you on the body. By using the your taiji skills you can render the opponent incapacitated. Chin Na must be applied quickly because the opponent can use anti-Chin Na techniques. The anti-Chin Na techniques will prevent you from applying Chin Na or gives the opponent a way to reverse and unlock the Chin Na technique.

Insight

For self defense it is good to learn Chin Na techniques after one learns Chansijin methods. Remember one needs to know Chin Na and how to reverse the Chin Na. Many martial styles external and internal uses Chin Na. there are more than one hundred types of Chin Na so do some research and practice then just like you practice push hands.

Meridians (TCM)

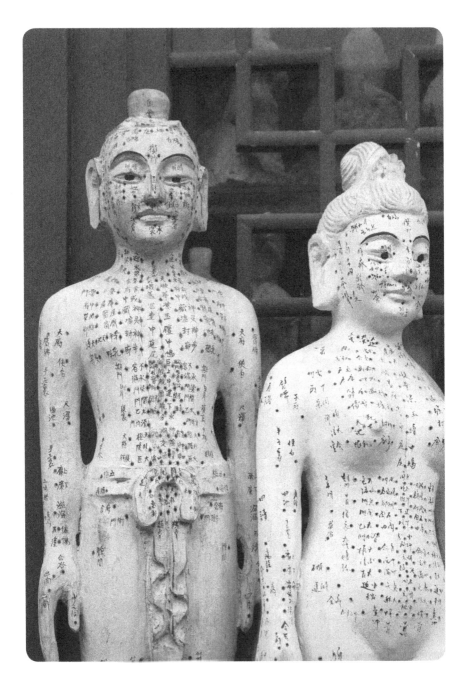

Understanding the Body System Structure

One must discuss the body system structure the same as one understands the structure of a building in order to understand Taijiquan, which involves not only Qi but includes the body and its internal systems.

The body has the following anatomy:

Skeleton
Brain
Spine and Spinal cord
Central and peripheral nervous system
Tendons and ligaments
Meridians
Breath
Muscles and more...

These above parts of the anatomy are connected together and work seamlessly in order for our body system to operate and function at an optimum performance. Whatever we do in life these systems work together to perform all of our operations. We cannot just assume by looking in the mirror that it is all there is. So as we practice our internal or external martial arts we must call upon these systems for function and success in our practice. Any malfunction affects our outcomes and performance. Once we go beyond the skeleton structure then we must move and conduct the following

- Responses
- Messages
- Blood
- Vital forces (energy)
- Fluids
- Oxygen

These different parts of the body system form a vast network that perfectly operates the body and its systems. All are utilized in our practice of Taiji and any internal martial art. One of those important networks that we must be aware is the blood and vital forces that move throughout the vast network within our body some call the jing luo or meridian system. This network is for carrying blood and vital forces to every part of our internal body system and consists of channels and acru-points similar to blood vessels which include arteries, veins and capillaries. These meridians also move vital forces such as Qi and blood throughout our system and this system has been identified and explained within the Traditional Chinese medicinal system. This system contains the pathways in which; blood, Qi (Qi), oxygen, fluids and nutrients travel to every part of the body. There are more than 365 acu-points within the body and there are twelve major channels that are associated with the zangfu organs that are the yin (zang) and the yang (fu) which include the following:

Zang

Lungs
Kidneys
Liver
Heart
Spleen

FU

Stomach
Gallbladder
Heart
Triple burner
Small intestine
Large intestine

All of these organs and their channels are stimulated when we practice our Taiji and internal postures. All moves when we move our bodies and the mind. Along with these meridians, organs, our muscles, tendons and ligaments also move as they are nourished by the blood and chi along with the marrow. Also there are eight extraordinary channels that are part of the matrix of channels and/or collaterals that assist us in a variety of ways that include healing and medical treatments. It is important to know this or understand as we progress in our practice and development of Qi, which consequently improves our health and longevity. Three major channels one must know is the Du Mai(督脉Back-governing vessel), Ren Mai(任脉Front-conception vessel), and Dai Mai (girding vessel, belt channel-waist) {usually we say Qijing bamai.} because they affect our movement of Qi around the entire body and they are called the microscopic orbit (小周天)

Microcosmic Orbit

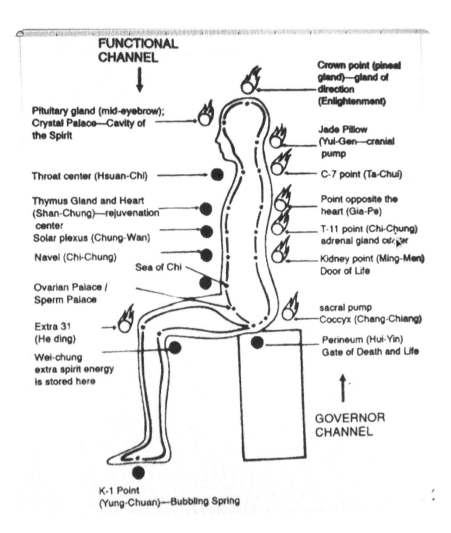

FUNCTIONAL CHANNEL

Crown point (pineal gland)—gland of direction (Enlightenment)

Pituitary gland (mid-eyebrow); Crystal Palace—Cavity of the Spirit

Jade Pillow (Yui-Gen—cranial pump

Throat center (Hsuan-Chi)

C-7 point (Ta-Chui)

Thymus Gland and Heart (Shan-Chung)—rejuvenation center

Point opposite the heart (Gia-Pe)

Solar plexus (Chung-Wan)

T-11 point (Chi-Chung) adrenal gland center

Navel (Chi-Chung)

Kidney point (Ming-Men) Door of Life

Sea of Chi

Ovarian Palace / Sperm Palace

Extra 31 (He ding)

sacral pump
Coccyx (Chang-Chiang)

Perineum (Hui-Yin)
Gate of Death and Life

Wei-chung extra spirit energy is stored here

GOVERNOR CHANNEL

K-1 Point (Yung-Chuan)—Bubbling Spring

Microcosmic Orbit

The purpose of the Microcosmic Orbit practice is to create a continuous circular energetic loop between what typically, in an adult human body, are two distinct meridians: the Ren Mai (Conception Vessel) and the Du Mai (Governing Vessel). There is also a macroscopic orbit (大周天) but more on that later and it's an advanced practice. This microcosmic orbit is a qigong practice so you should learn how to practice this easy Qigong exercise. One should practice the moving of energy via the microscopic orbit and eventually the macroscopic orbit. When you are doing your silk reeling or pole standing (zhanzhuang) you are practicing the movement of Qi via these internal meridians. This is incorporated within your internal Taiji or qigong practice, so don't skip understanding this vital information.

Seven Important Areas of the Universal Body

The body is a microcosm of the universe and it is important to understand this is similar to the stars in the universe. The important seven parts of the body in Taijiquan is:

Head
Shoulder
Elbow
Hand
Hip
Knees
Feet

We must know how these parts work separately, which is easy and how they work together as part of the unit body system in Taiji. Sounds quite simple, hint; can you pick up a hundred pound bag with one hand? Can you pick up a hundred pound chain with one hand? Does all your parts work together as one unit? Are you connected to the universe, the heavens and the earth, and nature? We are all part of the one universe. Which parts work together in pairs? First check the six harmonies.

Six Harmonies

Above is listed the body parts and now we must understand how the parts harmonize with each other. We cannot forget the six harmonies, which is vital for our practice. There are 3 external harmonies and 3 internal harmonies. The importance is that these extremities move together. The internal also move with the external. The harmonies, reminds us that if our hand and foot are not moving together or your elbow is past your knee they are not in total harmony.

External harmonies	Internal harmonies
Shoulder-hip	Mind-intention (yi)
Elbow-knee	Intention (yi)-Qi
Hand-foot	Qi-(body) breath
	Spirit-Qi
	Body-heart

This is important in Taiji and other internal martial arts such as Xingyi, Baqua and Liuhebafa (Water Style Boxing). Liuhebafa (Six Harmonies and Eight Methods) is a special internal martial art system passed down by Master Wu Yi-Hui.

Liuhebafa is an internal martial art that is a combination of Xingyi, Taiji and Baqua. The most important aspect of this system is one's mind and intention. In other words, one's intention should be sharply focused on each movement, and the movements are then led by one's mind and intention. Intention, rather than physical force, is used. One's intention, connects the postures, and makes them a seamless whole. That is one of the major keys of internal martial arts.

Eight Methods of Liuhebafa refer to (1) Qi (energy), circulating Qi to concentrate Shen (spirit); (2) Gu (bones), collecting energy inside the bones; (3) Xing (form), incorporating animal forms from nature; (4) Sui (to follow), circular and smooth motion responding to the situation; (5) Ti (lifting), lifting from the crown of one's head to have a floating feeling; (6) Huan (returning), coming and going in a cycle; (7) Le (suspending), being motionless and calm while waiting; and (8) Fu (concealing), looking for an opening while concealing yourself. Most internal styles focus on the philosophy of six harmonies and 8 methods.

Insight

This is important to understand as we practice we must insure that all of these internal systems are working at optimum and our circulation is open and smooth including blood, fluids and Qi. When we practice, part of our work is to dissolve previous injury blocks, areas of stasis, energetic blocks, slow circulation and choppy movement internally and externally as a part of our advancing in our practice. When you hear of blockages or reference to ice in joints or pains and stiffness it is part of our task to free up these problems and become smooth and free flowing in our practice of our postures and forms.

As we practice many of these problems will disappear. This information will help you understand when the body system is not functioning properly or you cannot explain why the blood or energy is not reaching a certain place or there are some functions you cannot accomplish until you are able to continue and release anything in these meridians that is slowing or impeding the process. For example let's say you cannot fajin, you then will realize that there is a problem you must overcome and this relates to the body system that must be corrected. Another example, you have no peng, then again you can refer it back to the body system. Now one must understand your body and its connection to the earth (yin) and the heaven (yang) internally is similar to the universe and so when all is interconnected you are like the micro universe. So your practice of Taiji and the movement of the mini universe is similar to the universe we experience everyday. Taiji and internal systems require knowledge of the medical internal systems on some level such as Traditional Chinese Medicine (TCM). If your hand is moving by itself then you are not in harmony so remember the harmonies.

For example: In keeping with TCM understanding and how it is important to Taiji there are important additional essential points we must keep in mind and be clear about:

- o Ni wan point on the top of the head to swallow heavens Yang Qi
- o Dantian and the lower dantian the storehouse of our Qi
- o Yungquan point based in the bottom of our feet called the bubbling brook connected to the Earth and where we draw in Yin Qi
- o Loa Gong point in the hand described as Buddha palm used to emit Qi used for healing or striking an opponent

Meditating on Wuji and the Internal Universe

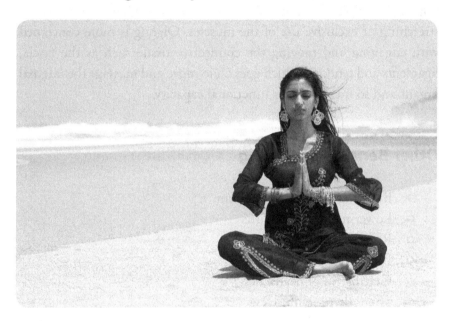

Qigong Training

Qigong can be translated as "energy work" and is a general term for gentle exercises, which are primarily aimed at gently opening the body, increasing physical awareness, increasing the circulation of fluids within the body (such as blood or lymph). It is a branch of traditional Chinese medicine (TCM), which originated from ancient medicinal practices of energetic practices and Taoism along with herbal medicine, bone setting and acupuncture.

Qigong is different than practices such as Yoga as Qigong is not about stretching or exclusive use of the muscles. Qigong is more concerned with engaging and moving the connective tissue such as the fascia, ligaments and tendons, which goes on to move and massage the internal organs and so increase their functional capacity.

Other Benefits of Qigong

- ○ Boosting the immune system,
- ○ Lowering blood pressure,
- ○ Reducing stress,
- ○ Boosting alertness,
- ○ Getting rid of headaches,
- ○ Strengthening muscles,
- ○ Increasing balance and flexibility,
- ○ Easing the effects of chronic illness,
- ○ Increasing lung capacity,
- ○ Improving disposition,
- ○ Improving pancreatic function, digestion and
- ○ Reducing stress on the heart.

Who Can Practice Qigong?

Everyone can practice Qigong forms There are forms for those who need to stand, remain seated or lay flat on a bed There are many different types of forms such as Zhanzhuang (standing pole), 8 Treasures (or Brocades), medical Qigong forms for treating various illnesses, Chansijing (silk reeling), hard and soft Qigong forms for martial arts.

Most standard Qigong forms can be done by just about anyone who can walk steadily for 20 minutes without pain or losing one's breath.

There are no special background or abilities required.

The movements are simple and easy to learn.

There are some contra-indications for Qigong:

- If you have or will be getting an organ transplant,
- If you have an active case of diarrhea,
- If you are taking an immuno-suppresive drug,
- If you have an untreated broken bone,
- If you are having a psychotic episode or event.

**Practicing Hunyuan Qigong with
Grandmaster Feng Zhiqiang in China**

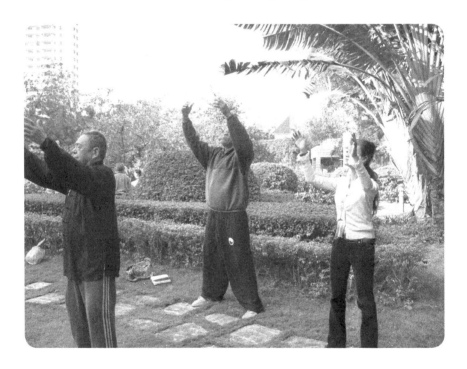

Zhanzuang Post Standing

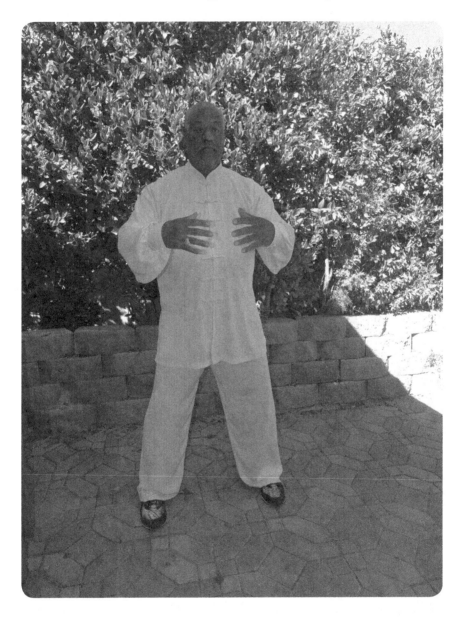

Zhanzuang Universal Post Standing

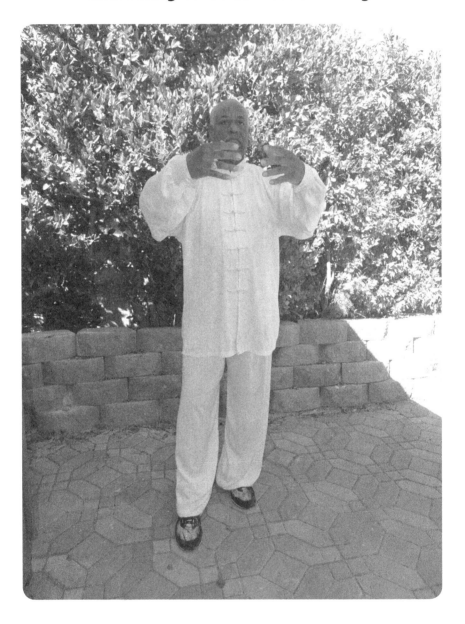

Gong or Kung Training

Gong (kung) training or some call kung is required for all those wishing to reach a high level in their practice of Taiji or any internal martial arts. The importance at an advanced level is the ability to increase the development and cultivation of energy and the ability to use the energy for health, healing and self defense. The higher-level skills require the Gong training, which is beyond just the practice for basic health or competition. It is up to you to train or seek out a teacher who can assist your gong training. But it should not be skipped over if you are seeking to become a master of Taiji or internal martial arts. For example, Taiji artists should do the microcosmic orbit meditation practice, which is the movement of Qi via the Governor (down the back of the body) and Conception (down the front of the body) meridians so that the energy can circulate through the body. This will help to clear any blockages in those channels and increase the flow of Qi. Clearing of blockages, also include the opening of the energy gates of the body to insure that the Qi can move smoothly throughout the body. These energy gates relate to the joints such as the neck, shoulders, elbows, wrists, hips, kua(胯) (relax), knees, ankles and feet. This also includes the energy passing through the mouth and the spine transversing the Du mai to the Ren mai and the Dai mai (belt channel.)

These energy gates must open and close and allow Qi to pass through freely and smoothly. A frozen shoulder joint will block Qi from moving just as the knee joints can block Qi from flowing to and form the yong quan (bubbling brook) point in the feet. It is important to loosen and relax the hips and kua(胯) so energy can flow up and down (sink) to the feet. So exercises such as making lots of circles, shaking and loosening the body and spiraling the joints helps to open these important energy gates along with your standing post practice.

The Dantians

As part of Qigong training one must also understand the dantians. There are three dantian. The dantian is called the energy elixir field. Energy is stored and flows through these dantian fields. The dantian fields are areas and not points. They work together to keep us healthy. The three dantians are as follows:

Upper dantian (上丹田, **Shang DanTian**)	Yin tang area: between the eyebrows	Spirit center-Yi	wisdom
Middle dantian (中丹田, **Zhong DanTian**)	Ren 17: area-heart area (middle of chest)	Qi center: post birth (**hou tian Qi**)	Love and compassion
Lower dantian (下丹田, **Xia DanTian**)	Ren 4: area 3 fingers below the naval	Essence: center-pre-birth (**xi tian Qi**)	Sexual energy, vitality and prowess

Insight

In China, it is very common to see people of all ages (from 4 years old to well *into their 90's!)* doing Qigong and Taiji every morning in the parks or even along the sidewalks or in front of their apartment buildings. Everyone is gracefully moving in slow motion. It is quite beautiful to watch. Qigong is practiced along with Taiji since Taiji is the practice of internal energy (neigong 内功). Qigong will help to heal any problems or stagnation in the internal system along with other Qigong healing methods. Qigong is utilized in a variety of ways to make martial artists stronger and immune to physical attacks such as hard Qigong. Also soft Qigong is utilized in order to increase Qi. As part of our practice we absorb Qi from the earth, heavens and universe so Qigong is an integral part of our practice of internal martial arts and longevity. As we practice dantian gong training, gathering Qi from the earth and the universe our

Qi will build and become stronger which we can use to heal ourselves, protect our own health and utilize it for martial arts. When practicing your Taiji focus your mind on the dantian to increase the flow of Qi in the dantian. The dantians is also connected to the breath as they work together. So breathing is important and should be normal, relaxed and in harmony with your practice of internal martial arts.

Master Golden Lai, and Author in Kowloon Park

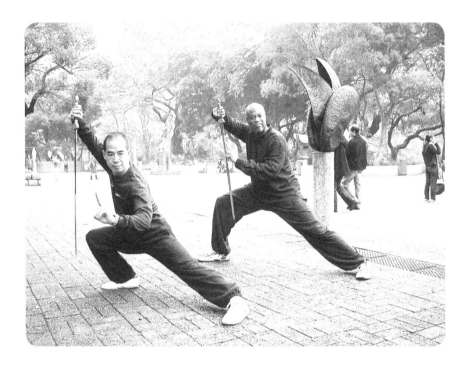

Training with Types of Weapons as an Extension

Training empty handed is the first requirement. After one reaches to a more advanced level it is important to practice with weapons. Proficiency in weapons should be a must and is for all martial artists who want to achieve a higher level of success. For internal practitioners, weapons assist in your development and advancement towards mastery so it is vital to practice with weapons in order to extend your practice beyond your short reach, and body. Keyword is extension. Variations of Taijiquan involving weapons also exist, such as Taijijian.

The weapons training and fencing applications employ:

- *Jiàn*剑 a straight sword, practiced as *Taijijian*;
- *dāo*刀, a saber, sometimes called a broadsword;
- *shàn* 扇, a folding fan, also called and practiced as *Taijishan*;
- *gùn*棍, a 2m long wooden staff and practiced as *Taijigun*;
- *Qiāng*枪, a 2-4m long spear.

More weapons still used by some traditional styles include:

- *pūdāo*扑刀, long-hilt broadsword;
- *Jǐ*戟, halberd;
- *mù zhàng*木杖, cane;
- *shéng biāo*绳镖, rope dart;
- *sānjié gùn*三节棍, three sectional staff;
- *fēng huǒ lún*风火轮, Wind and fire wheels;
- *biān*鞭, whip

Insight

The practice of weapons should not be taken lightly and should be practiced as one grows within their practice. Weapons are practiced two fold, one way is training on how to use weapons as a martial art and the second is the essential importance of utilizing weapons to extend beyond the self and the body. Weapons are considered long range as compared to the fist and body, which is considered short range. This also will help practitioners' ability to extend their mind-intent. Train as if the weapon is like your arm, not separate from it.

Training in the 13 Energies

What are the thirteen energies that one needs to train and perfect? The thirteen energies coordinate with the 13 Postures of Taiji. They are the foundation of Taijiquan. The 13 Postures form the basis of the martial art and push-hand skills. They were derived from the Eight Trigrams (the first 8 postures - energies) and the Five Elements. The postures are well known and must be taught, practiced, internalized not only as a physical move but also with mind-intent and understood that where the mind goes so does the energy. Below are the 13 energies as follows:

- *Peng*掤, ward-off
- *Lu*捋, (roll-back)
- *Ji* 挤, (press)
- *An*按, (push)
- *Cǎi*採, (pull-down)
- *Liè*挒, (split)
- *Zhǒu*肘, (elbow strike)
- *Kào* 靠, (shoulder strike)

These next 5 are derived from the five elements or 5 can be considered 5 directions

- Chin (advance)
- Tui (retreat)
- Ku (look left)

- Pan (look right)
- Ting (center)

Since the 13 postures are considered the chief principles of Taijiquan, the 13 principles are executed with mind intent, then, Qi will follow, along with the corresponding physical movement as one unit. This means that when the mind is focused on a specific area of the body, the Qi will flow into that area. When the Qi flows into an area, power will follow. Along with that flow of energy, the body must conform to the requirements so the Qi can flow unobstructed throughout or be diminished until there is only a small amount of force is expressed. So do not forget these points also discussed in the Classics.

- Sinking of Shoulders and Dropping of Elbows
- Relaxing of Chest and Rounding of Back
- Sinking Qi down to Dan Tien
- Sink the mind
- Lightly Pointing Up the Head
- Relaxation of Waist and Hip
- Differentiate Between Empty and Full: Yin and Yang
- Coordination of Upper and Lower Parts of the Body
- Using the Mind Instead of Force
- Harmony Between Internal and External
- Connecting the Mind and the Qi
- Find Stillness Within Movement
- Movement and Stillness Present at Once
- Continuity and Evenness Throughout the Form

As part of the classics the principles are to be memorized and internalized within your practice. So it is vital to go over the principles again and again until one gains the pearls enclosed. Once the basics are understood then the practitioner has to go deeper and understand more. So advanced advice and insight is imparted within the Classics such as *Expositions of Insights into the Practice of the Thirteen Postures*.

Expositions of Insights Into The Practice of The Thirteen Postures

(by Wu Yu-hsiang (Wu Yuxian) (1812 - 1880) sometimes attributed to Wang Chung-yueh as researched by Lee N. Scheele)

The hsin (mind-and-heart) mobilizes the Qi [vital life energy or Qi].

Make the Qi sink calmly; then the Qi gathers and permeates the bones.

The Qi mobilizes the body. Make it move smoothly, so that it may easily follows the hsin.

The I [mind-intention] and Qi must interchange agilely, then there is an excellence of roundness and smoothness. This is called "the interplay of insubstantial and substantial."

The hsin is the commander, the Qi the flag, and the waist the banner.

The waist is like the axle and the Qi is like the wheel.

The Qi is always nurtured without harm.

Let the ch'i (Qi) move as in a pearl with nine passages without breaks so that there is no part it cannot reach.

In moving the Qi sticks to the back and permeates the spine.

It is said "First in the hsin, then in the body."

The abdomen relaxes, then the Qi sinks into the bones.

The shen [spirit of vitality] is relaxed and the body calm.

The shen is always in the hsin.

Being able to breathe properly leads to agility.

The softest will then become the strongest.

When the Jing shen is raised, there is no fault of stagnancy and heaviness. This is called suspending the head top.

Inwardly make the shen firm, and outwardly exhibit calmness and peace.

Throughout the body, the Yi relies on the shen, not on the Qi. If it relied on the Qi, it would become stagnant.

If there is Qi, there is no li [external strength].

If not focused on Qi, there is pure steel.

The Jin [intrinsic strength] is sung [relaxed], but not sung; it is capable of great extension, but is not extended.

The Jin is broken, but the Yi is not.

The Jin is stored (having a surplus) by means of the curved.

The Jin is released by the back, and the steps follow the changes of the body.

The mobilization of the Jin is like refining steel a hundred times over. There is nothing hard it cannot destroy.

Store up the Jin like drawing a bow.

Mobilize the Jin like drawing silk from a cocoon.

Release the Jin like releasing the arrow.

To fa-jin [discharge energy], sink, relax completely, and aim in one direction!

In the curve seek the straight, store, then release.

Be still as a mountain, move like a great river.

The upright body must be stable and comfortable to be able to sustain an attack from any of the eight directions.

Walk like a cat.

Remember, when moving, there is no place that does not move. When still, there is no place that is not still.

First seek extension, then contraction; then it can be fine and subtle.

It is said if the opponent does not move, then I do not move. At the opponent's slightest move, I move first."

To withdraw is then to release, to release it is necessary to withdraw.

In discontinuity there is still continuity.

In advancing and returning there must be folding.

Going forward and back there must be changes.

The Form is like that of a falcon about to seize a rabbit, and the shen is like that of a cat about to catch a rat.

Changes caused by my opponent fill him with wonder.

Study the function of each posture carefully and with deliberation; to achieve the goal is very easy.

Pay attention to the waist at all times; completely relax the abdomen and the Qi rises up.

Insight

Above the *Exposition of Insights of the Thirteen Postures* tries to explain what is transpiring or what should be happening in our internal practice. It also expounds upon growth of the practitioner who can sense and realize the subtle movements within the postures that occur as the practitioner moves to the advanced level of their practice. This is the part of the gong training that we must be aware of and be sure that we are internally moving the Qi using the Yi and not the muscle or physical attributes of our self. The importance of the mind intent and the movement of the Qi is paramount and we must be totally aware of what we are doing or what we are not doing so we can be able to learn or correct ourselves. What we do not understand we can learn and/or question our Teacher or our own self.

The insight and *Song of the 13 Postures* will greatly help you in achieving growth in your practice. The importance of the classics is to help you to identify anything missing from your forms practice, assist you in your practice, your push hands skills, and your advancement to a higher level. If you feel something is not correct in your practice consult your Teacher and/or the classics.

Strength versus Power (Li versus Jin)

This point is vital as you grow within your training and your practice. Many Teachers will advise you correctly but if you have no teacher or you practice at home by yourself you must be clear on the use of Li (muscle strength) as compared to the use of internal jin or Qi (energy). When practicing your Taiji or any internal martial art the practitioner should focus on the movements by mind intent that will consequently move the Qi or jin and the body at the same time. When one first starts their practice a lot of the postures and movements are by utilizing Li strength (clumsy force). This will diminish over time if you follow the principles and what is outlined in the classics. As you grow with using mind intent the use of Li will diminish and then the internal energy Qi can move and circulate throughout the body. Refrain from using muscles and continue to use little or no muscle strength. This will help the flow of internal energy and minimize any energetic blockages. It will also assist you to develop springy (jin) power and you will be able to exhibit (jin) power when required. Many people ask the question how can you practice and not use muscles when performing martial arts forms such as Taiji.

The li utilized in Taiji is a conduit liken to lighting a bulb in your house. The light comes on without having to slap you with the wires but the wires are there in the wall. Another example, your car moves when you step on the gas. You don't see the gas igniting but you know and trust it will, if you turn on the engine. The car also turns the corner by you turning the steering wheel and you trust that when you turn the steering wheel the car wheels will turn and go around the corner. You don't have to get out the car to turn each wheel by hand. So remember the mind goes before the body moves, the Qi will move the body, the muscles stay relaxed and trust you will move accordantly.

Insight

Taiji like all internal martial arts means internal or inside. Be mindful of this. If a movement is purely physical without the mind intent, it is not Taiji. Which one comes first, the chicken or the egg? I say the mind intent to have chicken and eggs. This follows the principal of first the Void, then yin and yang were born, and separated then ten thousand things came into being only to return to the Void. Remember to relax the muscles. External styles focus on muscles and speed for their power, not Taijiquan. Taiji focuses on mind intent and internal energy to move the body.

Ponder the Circle

What are you thinking when you think circle? Is it really a circle? What do you think about when you try to determine if you are circular in all your movements? Do you think about the steering wheel of your car? Do you think that the waist is the commander and your waist is round? Do you contemplate the tires of the car or millet stone that makes the soy or rice milk by turning it round and round? Answer this question how many circles are in a circle. How many dimensions are in a ball? Have you become the ball? Have you done your math and understand the radius of a circle and the diameter of the circle within the ball? What is the center of a circle? Where are you in the circle? Enough with the questions, I can answer them but then you won't do your homework. The answers are within you. Do you understand the soft or hard ceaselessly changing within the circle. Do you move within and without of the circle no matter if going up or down or left or right. The ball always turns left and right, up and down.

Second Wushu and Taijiquan Conference in China

Happy

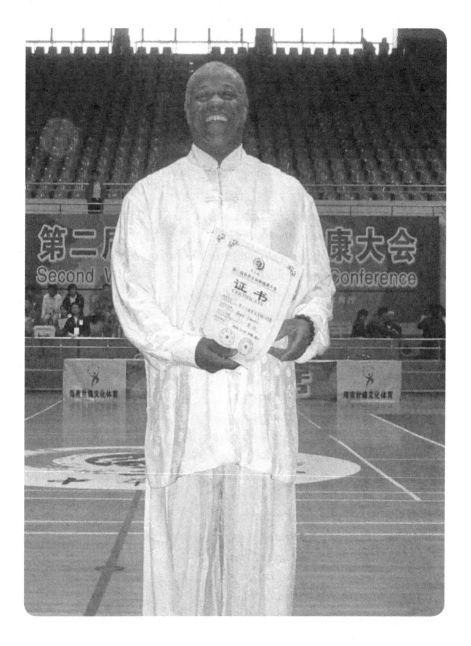

Qi (Chi)

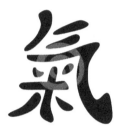

Song of Circulation of Qi
(from Lost Taiji Classics from the late Ching Dynasty (16 to 19 century) by Douglas Wile)

The QI is like the waters of the Yangtze
As it flows eastward wave upon wave;
Arising from the "bubbling well" point in the ball of the foot,
It travels up the spine in the back
Arriving at the ni-wan in the center of the brain
It returns to the yin-tang between the brows.
The mind leads the Qi
And never leaves it for an instant.
For example, if you want to raise your right hand
The mind QI first reaches the armpit,
Then following the kinetic energy,
You will feel the mind-QI in the pit of the elbow
Turning over your hand
The QI will arrive at the nei-kuan point on the inside of the arm above
the wrist,
If the right hand extends outward in push
The palm will slightly protrude
As the QI travels to the yin side of the hand
And finally reaches the tips of the fingers
It is the same with one or two hands
And the feet and hands arc no different
If I reveal one side to you

You should be able to complete the other three for yourself
If you practice in this way
Your whole body will be connected as if with a single thread
The mind leads the Qi
And the whole body moves as one
In movement, everything moves;
In stillness, all is still
In speed, all is fast
In slowness, all is slow
Exhale, concentrate your energy, and repel the opponent
Inhale, expand your energy, and return it to the dan-tien
Circulate the QI as if threading a pearl with nine beads
So that the whole body is thoroughly penetrated
But strictly avoid moving the Qi too rapidly
So that it jumps from the spine to the fingertips
It must touch every point step by step
And pass through each and every gate
It is essential that it move by the proper measure
and that the internal and external follow what is natural
If the mind and strength are harmonized
then after long practice, the QI will naturally pass through the gates.
In this way, after many years,
You will become an arhat of steel.

The mind and QI are rulers,
And the bones and flesh are ministers,
The waist and legs are commanders;
The hands are vanguards,
And the eyes and skin are spies.
The ruler gives orders and the ruler acts.
The spies must immediately report to the commander,
And the commander issues orders to the troops.
Ruler and follower work together;
Above and below act in harmony,
And the whole body is one flow of Qi.

Insight: Ponder Qi Circulation

Ponder Qi circulation and determine if your movements are simultaneously moving the Qi within our body system. We talk about movement, about postures and energies and all of this to make sure our internal Qi is also moving and circulating within our own systems through any blocks, tension, stress, injuries and anything mentally keeping us from relaxing and moving our Qi. If your Qi is not moving freely one must relax more, let go of tension, stress and insure our body posture is in the right position when we move within our forms. Another insight is to determine if one has frozen joints that need to loosen and open in order for Qi to move freely. So not only must we move freely our bodies but also our internal energy (Qi).

Also where is your Qi? Is your Qi sinking to the dantien or to the bottom of your feet. Is your breath sinking also? Are you relaxed enough so your breath and Qi can sink to the bottom of your feet. Once the Qi sinks to the bottom of your feet then it can move up and circulate throughout your system. Some people can feel their Qi moving but their Qi doesn't sink to the bottom of their feet for various reasons touched on above. Remember the mind must go to the bottom of your feet also. To start, get the Qi and breath to sink to the lower dantian. After that is accomplished sink the Qi to the feet.

Ponder the Stretch

If you practice any martial art whether it is external Wushu or any type of internal martial art including Taiji you must stretch your limbs and body. I have seen too many practitioners who don't stretch. Stretching will help your limbs and body to become more limber and help your circulation. If a runner wants to run track the runners must stretch and limber up. All players of any sport know they must stretch their body, which helps to also protect their joints, ligaments, muscles and tendons. As one advances in their practice of Taiji or martial arts also one should do power stretching to improve the flow of Qi and blood and help the body to become one unit. If you need to kick or punch then you need to stretch, but do not over stretch.

Two Taiji Practitioners

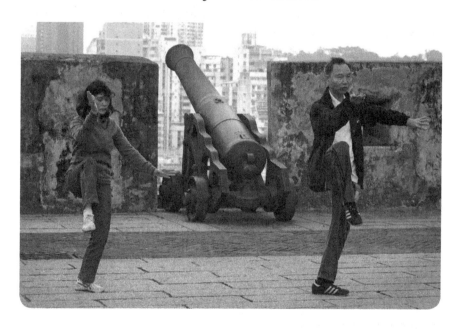

Mastering the Five Steps Wu Bu

Five Steps (5 Steps, Directions, Footwork Techniques, Movements) - Wu Bu

Nimble, responsive, and coordinated footwork is essential to success in all styles of martial arts. Taijiquan requires precise footwork and legwork. The placement and movement of the legs and feet as they relate to the powerful and coordinated application of energy in Taiji stances and postures in forms-work, drills, and push hands.

"In Chinese martial arts, Bu is a general term referring to stance and foot/leg work. If we keep in mind our general definition for the Shi San Shi or the 13 Powers, an ideal translation for WuBu might be something like: "powers based on the five stages of footwork" or, "the five implicit behaviors of the stance" or even (considering the interactive nature of the Wu Xing), "the five innate powers and conditions arising from the natural cycle of stages within the stance". It is the inherent behaviors, strengths and stages that are the subject in the WuBu, not the shape or position of the stance as such the innate conditions for power in stance work. We are also referring to the cyclical way in which these powers emerge and dissolve. Also, as importantly, we are speaking of the natural constraints inherent in the legwork." - (Sam Masich, Approaching Core Principles.)

"Wubu are the five footwork skills. Wu means five. Bu means step. In fact it is more about Shenfa - body movement skills because footwork and body movement have a very tight relationship. They should be combined together. It is said "the body follows steps to move and steps follow the body to change", "Body movement and footwork skills cannot be forgotten. If any of these is omitted, one does not need to waste his time practicing anymore." The body movement skills and footwork skills are about how to move the body in fighting. Only when the body can move to the right position (distance and angle), can the hand skills work well. Thus, it is said Wubu is the foundation of "Bafa."- Break Step, an Entering Forward Step.

Taijiquan does use front heel kicks, toe kicks, and jump kicks, sweeping kicks, and knee strikes. The Five Stepping Movements all primarily involve movements of the legs and feet, with little emphasis upon the arms or hands. When kicking, the arms are used to balance the body, facilitate the control, power, or speed of the kicks, and to have the arms in a defensive position. So it is important to associate kicking techniques with the Five Stepping Movements.

In Taijiquan practice, kicking is done slowly, effortlessly, gently, and smoothly; and considerable balance and strength are required to extend the legs fully, slowly, and in strict form. In external martial arts practice the kicks are done with much more speed and power. These are the Yin and Yang approaches to kicking, and are needed, by martial artists.

There are around 14 different stepping methods from Taijiquan. However, these are divided up into the main five methods of the step:

1. **Forward** (Jin bu-Element metal), Brush Knee and Twist Step
2. **Backward** (Tui bu- Element wood), Retreating Steps, Stances, and Looking Back Step Back and Repulse Monkey
3. **Look Left** (Ku- Element water), Parting the Wild Horse's Mane, Waving Hands Like Clouds, Strike the Tiger Deflect, Parry and Punch Single Whip
4. **Gaze Right** (Pan - Element fire) Parting the Wild Horse's Mane, Strike the Tiger Brush Knee, and Twist Step Slant Flying
5. **Central equilibrium** (Ding- Element earth) Zhong Ding

Golden Cock Stands on Right Leg - Left Knee Strike Golden Cock Stands on Left Leg - Right Knee Strike Needle at Sea Bottom Fair Lady Works the Shuttles

These 14 steps below are used for receiving and issuing Qi. These steps are utilized in Taiji boxing, both in push hands and in forms training. The steps are the root of the body. Flexibility comes from the knees. Your steps must be proper in order to demonstrate power and dexterity. So practice the proper stepping in Taijiquan.

1. Break Step: An entering forward step.

This step is one of the main stepping methods of Taijiquan. This step is found in mostly in Taiji. The front foot is placed down on its heel, then as the body moves forward, the toes are placed. However, the weight does not come any more forward than the middle of the foot. The thighs and knees are curved and collecting while the rear thigh is less curved than the front. We never retreat in Taijiquan and we can do this because of this stepping method. The rear foot controls the waist in yielding and throwing away the attacker's strength. The waist is controlled during this step by the rear foot. There is an old Taijiquan saying: "To enter is to be born while to retreat is to die". So we never retreat, we rely upon the rear leg controlling the waist for our power and evasiveness without moving backward. The hands have Peng Jing. It is easy to revolve in this step as the toes come up with the revolving done on the heel while when contracting and issuing force, the toes touch the ground. A posture that uses this method is, Brush Knee and Twist Step.

2. Backward Break Step: A Move Backward Step.

This backward step is only used in the posture known as 'Step back & repulse Monkey'. The toes settle first followed by the heel with the waist being controlled this time by the front leg.

3. Rolling Step: A Looking Left Step.

Revolving left and right the foot sticks to the ground when you turn it to follow what the body is doing and in accordance with what the opponent is doing. This creates friction and can be used to gain energy. Using this stepping method, we do not have to lean forward or backward to move. The weight is placed upon the heel and the foot is concave as it is rolled to the left or right depending upon which foot is forward. The postures such as: 'Step Up, Parry & Punch', 'Hit Tiger Left & Right', and the movement just after 'Inspect The Horse's Mouth' all use this stepping method. This step along with the break step is the foundation of Taijiquan stepping and footwork. If a student finds difficulty in moving when the weight is placed onto the moving foot, then the 'rolling step' has not as yet been mastered. It should impart an easy and comfortable way in which to move.

4. Rising Step: An Equilibrium Step.

This step uses the power of one leg rising to cause the body to rise such as in Golden Cock Stands on One Leg. It trains the upper thigh's Peng jing and the thigh must move in a circular manner such as when lifting the right leg, the left leg must move in a clockwise direction in order to gain the fajing necessary for this movement.

5. Sinking Step: A Central Equilibrium Step.

This movement trains the lower thigh Peng jing and is used when the leg is lifted up and placed down while moving the body weight downward. The thigh does a circular movement the opposite of the above. So when performing Needle At Sea Bottom from the Old Yang Style, the right thigh does a counter clockwise circle keeping the backbone vertical. Also this is Chen's intercepting step.

6. Withdrawing Step: A Looking Left Step. It can also be called a Looking Right Step.

This step moves from 'inside to outside'. The thigh makes a circular movement in the case of Ride The Tiger back To Mountain, from the

Old Yang Style, the right thigh will do a clockwise circle in order to give the left palm great power. The eyes look firstly to the right then to the left.

7. Gathering Step: A Looking Left or gazing Right Step.

This step is done from outside to inside as in Wave Hands Like Clouds from Yang Style, the cross-stepping method. The hands and legs must have Lu Jing. The feet must move constantly stepping effortlessly. The 'gathering' is when the whole body is twisted when one foot goes behind the other. The right toe is placed first, followed by the heel as this can be the releasing of the Qi after the gathering.

8. Curved Step: A Looking Left or gazing Right Step

This is that step such as in Parting Wild Horse's Mane. It is called an 'outside drawing of silk method' as the leg attacks in a curve from the outside of the opponent's body as in a kind of sweep to his legs as the hands also attack. It is used for both attack and defense.

9. Slant Step: A Looking Left & Gaze Right Step

This step is taken to the corners diagonally such as in any other corner steps but more importantly Slanting Flying. The balance and timing must be perfect so that the step can step forward or backward at any time without hesitation.

10. Horse Riding Step: A Central Equilibrium Step.

This step such as in Single Whip when the rear leg is also sunk but not as much as the front and Fair Lady Works Shuttles, The weight is sunk onto both legs with slightly more weight being placed onto the front leg. Because of the controlling factor of the front or rear leg, it is said to have double Peng jing whereby the legs are in constant push and pull mode. I call this having the engine in idle ready to go.

11. Fishing Step: A Central Equilibrium Step.

This step moves to left or right as in the normal way of performing Wave Hands Like Clouds. The feet move directly to either side and the thighs must circulate, the left thigh makes a clockwise circle while the right one does a clockwise circle.

12. Fairy Step: A Central Equilibrium Step.

This step is when the point of the toe is placed onto the ground but is insubstantial. There is a rotation of the right thigh counter clockwise and a very slight lifting of the upper body and then a sinking.

13. Turning the Body over Step: A Looking Left and gazing Right Step.

This involves fajing so the spine is the main factor in this step. It is placed into such a position as to gain much power for a downward hammer fist to his arms followed by a chopping hand strike to vital points. The power is gained when the spine turns violently right to left to right. The thighs must be in control mode as in outward and inward drawing of silk so that the spine remains vertical to issue the power.

14. Push Step: Move/Enter Forward Step.

The rear foot follows the turning action of the front foot so that the body ends up facing 90 degrees to the right or left as in Apparent Close Up. The front foot (left usually) pushes the energy over to the right as the rear foot moves in accordance with what the front foot is doing. The pushing motion is necessary because of the martial application of this movement. The front foot contains Peng jing energy.

It is important to know that all steps must contain Peng jing and have central equilibrium. This is why we practice form, to learn about the stepping methods and how to perform them effortlessly and without thinking about them. The body moves in accordance with what the attacker is doing to us, so there is never a time when we will make an incorrect step. The stepping methods are there so that we can move quickly, releasing power as we move quickly, sinking as we lift and releasing as we gather. These methods are in other internal martial art styles such as other than Baguazhang and Xingyiquan.

Insights

Moving and stepping is all about yin and yang, insubstantial and substantial, and the applications of the internal martial arts. How to move, step, stay centered, maintaining ones equilibrium is about function and how one can apply the art. The stepping method of Taijiquan means the natural manner of stepping. Once you understand about central equilibrium, rooting and lightness and heaviness, then your timing will be perfect. This is why we practice the form, to learn about the stepping methods and how to perform them effortlessly and without thinking about them. The stepping methods are there so that we can move quickly, releasing power as we move quickly, sinking as we lift and releasing as we gather. Again remember peng jin and central equilibrium is everywhere.

Remember Taiji is a martial art not an aerobic activity or dance. Learning to do basic martial arts techniques is required. How to punch, kick, step, move, defend and attack is part of your martial arts training. Each posture is normally several applications. Even if you only learn one application for each posture one should know how to apply the basic thirteen energies or techniques, how to step and how to execute a proper (Taiji) punch or a kick.

Group practicing Yang Style Taiji

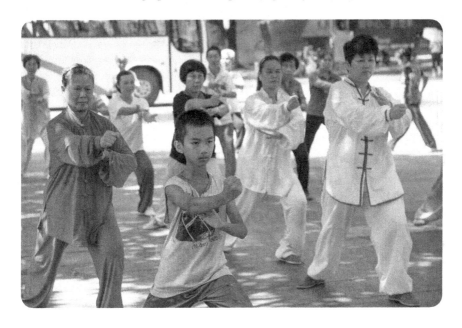

III

THE PATIENCE
(Dong Jin)

Practice Correctly

In order to practice correctly one has to understand fully what that means since we all think we practice correctly. So we must answer several questions in order to insure that we are practicing correctly so what does this mean for example:

When you move are you using mind-intent (xin-yi)?
Are you relaxed and /or Song?
Are you using brute force (Li) or Qi?
Are you standing tall and centered?
Are you using the waist or upper body?
Are you clear each time you move about substantial and insubstantial?
Is your breath normal or deep or are you breathing shallow?
Do you hold your breath?
Do you have tension?
Is your energy circulating smoothly?
Are you rooted all the time?
Are you sensing or pushing hands?
What direction are you moving?
Are you clear on what is yin or yang at any given moment in time?
Are you doing linear movement or circular movements?
Is everything moving as one unit?
Is everything moving in unison?
Do you have peng jin?
Are you balanced?
Are you following the principles of the classics?
Are you connected to the source?
Are you alive?

Insight

Above are a few questions that one should answer or contemplate while doing their practice. They touch upon areas we must consider to insure we are incorporating all of the principles and can demonstrate them. As we practice we will touch upon these essential points. As we correct and perfect our postures and our movement we will be right on course towards perfection. If there are questions you cannot answer then you eventually will learn the answers by doing your research.

Taiji Practitioners Performing

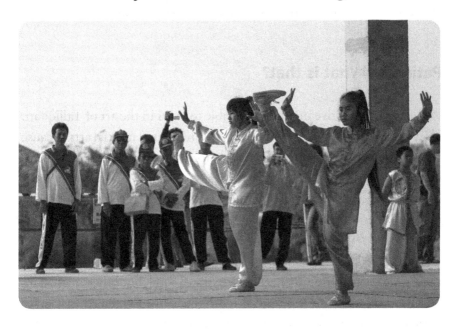

Practice makes Perfect

Practice is imperative and the frequency of that practice is up to you. One can practice once a week, three times a week or every day. It is up to you but remember if one wants to master anything one must practice to become familiar then practice to become highly skilled then practice more to become an expert. There are no substitutes, your Teacher cannot do it for you, smile. What goes along with major practice to reach some level of expertise is patience and perseverance.

Patience: What is that?

Patience is imperative in order to be able to excel in the art of Taijiquan. How can one be patient? It is the only way in internal martial arts because it is different than other external style forms due to the importance of relaxing and internalizing the energies, the ability for the Qi to soak into the bones and grow. This is why one cannot solve the solution in one day, one week, one month or one year.

One cannot skip high school and then go to college so one has to take their time to improve slowly. This frustrates some but others realize it's like waiting at the corner for the red light to turn green. It just takes patience. Some people bump around looking and seeking the quick answer to success or the quick secret knowledge that will make them an instant success but wind up realizing it takes training, practice and then patience. There are valid reasons for the utilization of patience because that too becomes a part of the internal practice of relaxation. We realize we cannot skip over the importance of patience. When you hear the words relax and to be Song (sung) and patient, it is for your own benefit. Another reason comes from one of the three faults we must not forget which are number three: "The third fault is impatience" (refer to the previous chapter: *Three Faults*).

Insight

Practice and patience go hand in hand. Taiji like other internal martial arts takes time and patience to build up and grow to a high level. Without patience many quit when they may on the brink of success right at the door. Taiji is liken to everyday life where many times some people quit because they lack the patience to preserve through the tough, the rough, the bitter, so progress, mistakes to corrections, lack of a qualified teacher, and lack of study. These things should not deter you from your practice of Taiji or your goal of mastery of the art. Even if you quit or stop for a while, even for years you can start over and continue until you reach the pinnacle of the success you are seeking.

First of all you probably know that Taiji is not a couple of years practice and so you must be in it for the long haul. Some say it takes a minimum of ten years. If you don't have the right teacher seek another teacher. If you don't know the classics, acquire them, read and study them. If you don't understand certain things ask your teacher or another practitioner. It is important to share with others on the same path. Don't be afraid to ask your teacher that is why they are there. Many teachers say the students do not ask any questions so they assume you got it, and do not need assistance or answers to the questions you are contemplating. Building internal energy takes time. It is a cumulative process. Being able to relax takes time. Using mind intent to move the body and deliver power takes time. It's all about the three Ps; practice, patience and perseverance.

Part of patience is included in your practicing and being mindful of what you are doing. Don't practice mindlessly. Think about what you are doing internally and externally. Such as learning the postures, relaxing as you practice, developing Qi as the mind move the Qi, learning to put it all together, and moving like one unit as all of this is happening at the same time, and knowing how each posture functions. All of this takes time to get to a place where it is effortlessly, smooth and one is Song: relaxed and rooted properly. If you are already doing all of this great!

There Are No Secrets

(The only secret is that there is no secret, ha.)

There are secrets. What are the secrets? The secret refers to the fact that many Teachers or Masters teach only quan (forms) and not the gong (internal training and development of jin), which is the most important part unless you are family or a special indoor disciple. The other secret is learning the applications. Also, there are very advanced skills many students are not ready or prepared to learn, and if learned may hurt themselves or other practitioners. Other than that there are not too many secrets.

Don't let that stop you, keep training and seeking the right teacher who will share his gong and higher skills training. The classics assure one that the secrets are hidden but almost in plain sight. We know that many teachers and Masters keep things from students many times especially if they are not disciples or inner door students. There are many reasons for that and we cannot fight about it, but most of all what you need to know is right in front of you. One has to do their own research and also listen carefully to their teacher who many times will reveal pearls that we let go right by us thinking it's not important or that valuable. Also there is a lot of material written on the subject so one should go to the library, and bookstore to acquire the materials to educate oneself on what is needed to grow their practice. Sometimes what we think is missing is written somewhere and we have not studied or applied it to our practice. Sometimes also teachers will hold back certain knowledge, why?

- student is not ready,
- student is not serious,
- student does not have good character,
- student cannot perform at that level or complete the tasks required,
- reserved for indoor students and disciples or family
- very few masters are teaching those skills

Insight

It's easy to blame the teacher but one should search themselves first. Also many teachers do not have the knowledge one seeks and so they are not to blame if they were never taught that particular knowledge or skill by their teacher. Some teachers want you to prove you are worthy of certain information. Don't fret over it, do continue to seek the information. No one will stop us from seeking advanced knowledge or skills. If we sincerely seek what we want to know, Do your homework. Do your own gong training such as Zhanzhuang or Qigong. I had a Teacher who told me that his training was for health and he was not taught the applications. He was honest and I was ok with it and continued to learn from him all he would share. It did not stop me from learning!

Importance of Practicing Patience

Imagine that when you are on the corner waiting for the light to change you become impatient waiting for the light to turn so you can cross the street. Instead you run in between the cars and traffic to get to the other side luckily you arrive on the other side safety just as the light turns green and the walk sign comes on for everybody else to cross. Instead of crossing before the walk sign you could of practiced your patience and waited then crossed safely with everyone else. Being patient is also a practice. First in learning, second in practice and third being patient and preserving until you develop a level of mastery. This is also part of your cultivation of your consciousness. Relaxation, calmness goes hand in hand with patience. Many martial artists want to succeed and become masters in the art but some do not only because they do not have the patience. Many masters of the art talk of reaching a level of being of Taiji consciousness, which takes training, practice and patience. They do not tell you once inside the door, that it's a door to a mansion of internal martial arts. No belt can be awarded to insure you are a master or have reached a high level of mastery. Belts are ok for show in internal martial arts as it is a personal practice requiring one to know their own self. This includes strengths, weaknesses and what one has accomplished, and what one needs to accomplish to reach their goal. Only through practice and patience can one reach a high level liken to the growing of a rose or a great oak tree. This also includes having a capable Teacher guiding you at the same time. This is where patience applies to the Teacher also.

Many people want the Teacher to reveal some secret antidote or move that will make you an instant master also but fortunately there is none and you have to do the work yourself in order to achieve a high level of mastery. Even when learning from the highest master one must practice, persevere and be patient as the Teacher explains and imparts important knowledge. Many teachers impart their knowledge one step at a time.

I had a Teacher who would tell me every time I came to train with him that he had taught me everything he knew. Then he would say ok lets learn something new. When he would say he had nothing new to teach me I would say nothing and patiently practice until my Teacher would present something new. This happened every time I saw him so I never asked for anything new just patiently abided my time, practiced and waited for whatever the Teacher would care to present and share with me. My patience helped me not only learn more but helped me to understand what I was learning, misunderstanding and/or missing from my practice. Remember simple things like developing your root or developing Qi, peng jin and/or becoming song require patience. So where do we go from here?

Back to Basics

Back to basics is one of the reasons one has to be very patient. One of the problems of learning internal martial arts such as Taiji we always think we know it all until we find out we do not or we know it in our heads but cannot produce the desired outcome when tested. I have found that one of the reasons is because it takes a long time to be able to show our skills we have learned and trained for. Competition is one venue but once one goes beyond that, one needs additional training and vital feedback. We do not want to give up or become dejected or feel short changed so one of the best things to do is to go back to the basics or reread the classics and check, recheck to see what we are doing right and what we are doing wrong or just not doing so we can revise, and move forward to the next level. When you meet masters of the art you realize quickly that you must continue to go back to the basics or classics until we ourselves have mastered the skills and techniques, and can show what we have mastered. This all requires a level of patience and one has to rise to the understanding that we must be patient and persevere until success. Refocusing takes time, practicing such things as "when one part moves all moves and when one part stops all parts stop." It may sound simple but not so simple, it takes practice and patience in order to do this. Practicing slowly is required and that takes patience but is rewarding if you do just that.

Lesson of Being Song (Relaxed)

Part of Taiji practice is developing Song within our training and it takes a long time. Everyone understands the word Relax but ask any ten people and the meaning would change. But why does the Teacher keep saying relax? Why does the classics say relax? This is one of the most important points and tenets of Taiji and all internal martial arts, why? One must be able to relax until Qi can flow uninhibited throughout the body and one can draw Qi from Nature and circulate it throughout the body. This is not a simple task. This requires one to relax but one of the most important tasks is to relax until one has reached a certain level of relaxation called Song.

What level of Song are you? Are you Fang Song? What does Fang Song mean? Fang Song means that you are relaxed, sunk, and have let go of all tension in the body and mind. This is a great dilemma because many practitioners ponder this question. Many practitioners think, I am relaxed but are they? Most teachers will say yes but you are not relaxed enough. When is relaxed enough? Song also includes your level of calmness within. One must be patient until they reach a certain level of Song and continue because there are many levels of Song. Also one has to be Fang Song in many places such as:

Body
The body must be relaxed, free of tension but not spaghetti

Mind
Mind must be calm, relaxed, clear, focused, and intentional

Joints
Joints must be relaxed and loose

Muscles
Muscles must be relax and free of needless tension

Tendons
Tendons must be relaxed, loose and flexible

Shen
Shen must be awake, alive,

Qi
Qi energy must be full, concentrated, settled, and flowing

Central equilibrium
One must become centered, calm and understand the importance of central axis

Insight

All of these important tasks and points require one to be Song (relaxed), not agitated or tense or over excited. In order to get to this level one must be Fang Song. Exactly what state or level that is one will know upon reaching that station in their practice. It takes practice as well as patience, always thinking I must relax until I am Song. Being Fang Song is the path to rooting along with mentally sinking into the ground, and it will assist with the Qi sinking into the bones. When your teacher says, you have to relax you will understand that you are not totally there yet. The concept of Fang Song will always be forefront in your training, practice, and in push hands practice. If you think you are already Song compare that to the lake when the water is still and see if it fits the above criteria. Until then relax and eventually you will become Fang Song. Remember water seeks its own level.

Remember Fang Song also implies that one is totally calm, relaxed, rooted, ready, agile, focused, flexible, confident, hips open, shoulders relaxed and settled and prepared for whatever comes your way. Water is always ready and can defend, encompass, deflect, accept, cover and move easily in any direction. When practicing push hands this philosophy of Fang Song will emerge as a test of your level of Song. Water flows unobstructed through a hose if there are no blocks or obstructions of any kind.

Being Song or Fang Song is vital because without it you cannot sink or become sunk in the body and mind. This will reveal a problem that needs to be corrected or healed. First, one must find the cause of why you cannot become Song. Here are some causes:

Mental tension (Stress, worry)
Physical tension
Psychological issues
Lack of sleep

Lack of joint looseness and flexibility
Blocked meridians
Blocked energy
Blocked circulation
Physical Structure
Physical ailments
New to practicing Song
Not letting go
Relying on muscles (Li-clumsy force)
Cannot relax tor sink the mind

These causes are clues that need to be explored in order to become Song if you are trying but not succeeding. So check each one and if one of them is the cause begin to correct, and remove the cause so you can become more relaxed and Song. Becoming Song will also help you to heal yourself of problems you may be having that are due to one of the above causes. Continue to practice becoming Song, being patient until you reach the level of Fang Song. Mentally repeat the verse 'weight balanced, mind balanced, listen behind, qi balanced in the dantien" when practicing your forms or standing post.

Why Patience?

Patience will help you realize your goals as an end result. Patience also cultivates discipline at the same time. If your goal is to reach a level of mastery then one must know when they have reached certain levels such as:

- You have learned the forms and feel comfortable and relaxed in your practice.
- One can show certain techniques and can do basic push hands. You are developing listening skill (ting jin).
- One has developed a root, some peng jin energy and can use it instead of zhouli (拙力raw force) energy.

- One can neutralize using peng jin, and the other seven energies.
- One can neutralize and discharge energy during push hands and can move 1000 pounds using 4 ounces.
- One can neutralize with any part of their body and discharge their opponents no matter what they do or try sensing the weaknesses of opponents.
- One has reached the stage of mastery and art and can do anything they want (Dong jin). "I know all about him but he knows nothing about me." I know me and I know him. (知己知彼，百战百胜，KNOW THYSELF,EVER VICTORIOUS)

Insight

When you have identified where you are in your development you can then reach for the next level or milestone until you have reached the level of mastery and art. If you feel stuck at any point seek help from a teacher, Master, or fellow practitioner and do more research. These steps are a way to determine if and when you have progressed so one does not just stay at the same level their entire life unless that is what they want. Also internal means internal and one has to be patient and mindful that they are doing an internal practice and not an external practice. Some students after much practice and thought, discover that they are losing power when they move and when they try to strike. They may have a strong shoulder or a big punch, but it is segmented and not part of a unitary body effort. This is because they have no root. So they must contine to be patient and continse to practice until they develop a root.

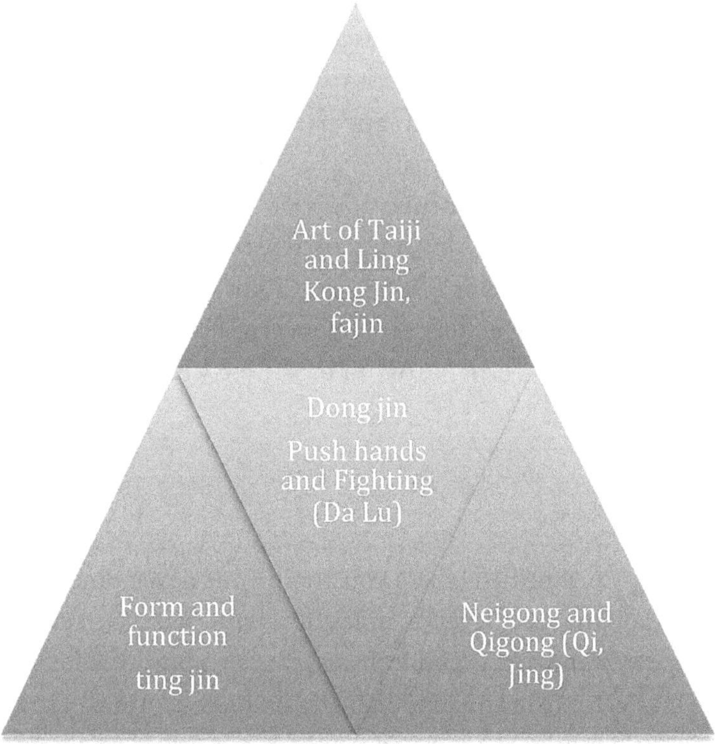
Art of Taiji and Ling Kong Jin, fajin
Dong jin
Push hands and Fighting (Da Lu)
Form and function
ting jin
Neigong and Qigong (Qi, Jing)

Patience and Perseverance of Qi, Jing and Fajin, Dong jin and Ling Kong jin

What in our Practice requires Patience and Perseverance?

Developing Peng Jin
Cultivating Qi then Jing
Cultivating Ting Jin
Learning Push Hands and Applications
Develop Dong Jin
Developing Fa Jin
Cultivating Higher Consciousness
Cultivating Ling Kong Jin

Listed above are the characteristics and skills that we must patiently cultivate through much practice, patience and perseverance. What does all this mean? Using patience and perseverance will help us to build strong Qi, to improve our overall health and then using the Jing to support the eight jins, and help us have the ability to be able to fajin in the future. The higher skills of Taiji, requires one to have strong Qi along with stronger mental intent. The next requirement is for the student to be able to sink their Qi to the dantian then to the bottom of the feet. The problem is that none of this happens fast as one would hope because it takes time to relax, practice, and a lot of patience. Any changes or corrections in the body and mind will have to happen first; such as any mental or energetic blocks, joints loosening, tension and stresses removed. Then as we reach a state of relaxation, rooting, developing sensitivity (ting jin), we can accomplish higher-level techniques such as spiral jing, spring jing, anti-locking (inside) jing, grasping jing, folding jing, applied (outside) jing, hidden jing, wave jing and shaking jing and the release of power called fajin. Once we understand the essence of neutralization and power called dong jin (he moves first, I arrive first), yielding and neutralizing, we can learn to exhibit and express high level skills and eventually with perseverance, be able to move opponents expressing high level techniques such as Ling Kong Jin. This comes with the cultivation and refinement of our consciousness that will change as we change so that we can progress to higher levels.

Insight

Everything is connected to Qi, Jin, the heart-mind (Xin-Yi), and Shen including the physical body as our internal practice. When learning the forms one is told to practice them slowly as to not miss anything and to give the practice time to internalize and to insure one is doing them correctly. It also assists you in developing mindfulness, and not the miss subtle interactions that are sensed as we practice. There are minute actions that can only be witnessed by practicing very slowly. This is part of your gong training, which is vital to cultivate Qi and will bear the fruits of your advancement to a higher level. With this patience and perseverance is required in order to cultivate the final essence of Taiji along with higher consciousness.

Remember Jing creates the body, Qi moves the body, Shen神 moves energy. One of the most important reasons to be patient is that as we practice over time we will begin to melt the ice in our joints, melt blocks, turn the ice into water, move our Qi and blood smoothly, breathe more deeply and then eventually turn the water into steam. This is all on the path to mastery so it is one of the rewards of practice, patience and perseverance. This all might seem a lot for a beginner but as one becomes advanced they will understand and be ready practice higher-level skills. At the same time we are changing our understanding of ourselves and the universe we live in. This is the change we experience within our own consciousness. This is the change that happens to, not only our own body system, it our mind, and energy. One cannot practice higher-level skills without neigong and corresponding changes in consciousness at the same time. So let us review the different levels of progression within our practice.

Training with Grandmaster Chen Zhenglei

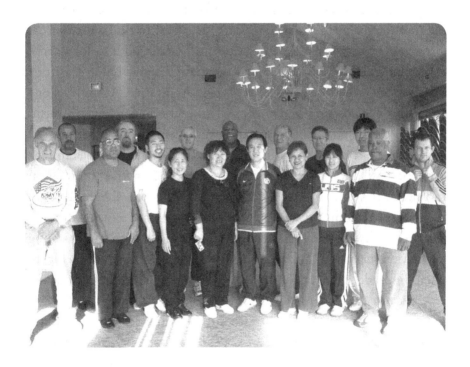

Insight: Into Four Levels of Progression within our Personal Practice

What are the four levels?

(1) Beginner

At the beginner level one is concerned about finding a teacher or good video of the forms they desire to learn. It is best to find a teacher. At this level one may try different styles until one decides to focus on a particular style of Taiji. This may eventually change but at least one has chosen a style, for example, let's say its Yang style. At his level one is learning the postures in the form whether it is a long or short form. This for some tends to be physical movements like any other martial art. But at this point of learning the form one should become familiar with the basic principles of Taiji along with the physical foundation and begin to learn to relax. In order to do this one should learn to become quiet, calm and the best way is to begin with basic meditation practices such as those associated with sitting meditation, and standing meditation such as zhanzhuang (post standing). This will begin to teach the student inner training that must be done for internal martial arts. Because the starting posture is in Wuji let us start there and begin to relax, calm down, let go of tension in the joints, body and mind. This will increase our awareness of ourselves internally and externally. Then as we begin to practice the different postures, we slowly relax, become aware of our body and how it moves, our structure, spine, head, limbs and our core.

We must practice our postures slowly and try to relax at the same time. Also try to relax within your movements by relaxing the muscles trying to not actively use any muscles. This is why we move slowly so we can become aware of what we are doing externally and internally. Remember we have a lot of limbs and parts of the body to move and also the internal such as Qi, blood, fluids along with the internal organs and the mind. One we learn the form, become more comfortable and feel our foundation is correct according to the classics and/or our teacher we continue to practice until we are comfortable and feel we can practice without supervision or thinking about every move. This takes time. We are now at the advanced beginner stage and are moving forward. What do you focus on besides the basic postures? We focus on being mindful of incorporating the following criteria: lightness, slowness, roundness, and evenness. We ask ourselves am I doing the posture correctly? After lots of practice we begin to remember the postures and practice to internalize them within our memory system.

(2) Intermediate level

When we progress to the intermediate level our practice is well underway and we feel confident about the postures of the form(s) and have them memorized and now are just relaxing and doing the postures, and feel we are doing Taiji. At this point we are still structural and concerned about how the postures look and feel and that they conform to our teachers direction or the video we are copying. We begin to learn the internal aspects of Taiji practice. We then begin to practice our meditation more especially standing post or universal standing post. We should be doing some sitting meditation such as microcosmic orbit and are relaxed enough to begin to soften up our minds and joints in order to relax more as we begin to feel the dantian, and then our feet and then the earth. We are standing more than 15 minutes and now can stand 30 minutes or more at a time progressing up to an hour. Our form is now standing to take shape and a feeling of roundness is emerging and a feeling of inner energy movement is appearing. At this point we are trying to correct our movements, our structure, the postures and learning that how we move (transition from one posture to the next) is more important than just moving. As our structure appears to be ok we then can begin to focus on what we are experiencing within our internal system. The intermediate level is a transition point to becoming more internal in our practice. For some they are focused on the correction and perfection of the forms for competition and this is ok. This should pass after a while once we have won several medals and trophies. Then back to our inner practice, which is more focused on the internal shape as opposed to the outer impression of our expression of the art of Taiji. At this level we now can begin to feel the difference between using Li and using mind intent to lead the Qi while we continue to relax the muscles more and more. At this point we become more aware of our breathe, our ability to relax the joints to turn them from ice to water by melting them and our heart/minds (xin-yi) leading us in our practice. This point is crucial to let the mind intent (xin-yi) to lead and that we relax our muscles as much as possible. At this point correction and testing is required to see if we are in compliance with the classics or what our teacher is teaching us. We have to be mindful of what we are doing or not doing as we practice.

Again at this crucial point we want to now emulate the silk worm and become connected within, leading our mind intent and inner Qi flow from one posture to the other to become very smooth and relaxed. An important note: do not focus on the Qi but on just being relaxed. At the same time check for the little nuances that seem to appear and require us to correct these minor mistakes. If we are feeling aches and pains we need to seek the cause of these and correct them. We need to understand our limitations and what we are doing correctly and what we are not. This is vital otherwise we may think we are progressing but may not be. This is a point where the Taiji teacher will need to guide us on the correct path but if we are alone at home we must guide ourselves by studying the classics and reflecting on what seems or feels correct, and testing what we are feeling or sensing. At this point it is good to have a teacher or friend test such things as the stance, movement, how relaxed are you, are you rooted, balance and give vital feedback. We can read the classics and check to see if we are following the principles outlined in the classics such as your head in its proper position, you rooted, you are using mind intent or are you still letting the body lead you, and etc.

Ask yourself if you feel your postures are connected without breaks in between. Some questions will pop up such as:

- Is the internal leading and the external following?
- Are you being patient.
- Are you practicing enough?
- Are you feeling more relaxed, more flexible,
- Are you feeling happy with your practice.
- Are you thinking good and positive thoughts?
- Am I following the principles correctly?

These questions are important and you can correct your thinking which will also correct your practice. Do you feel you are now doing internal practice or are you 60/40; 70/30; or 50/50 in terms of external to internal in your practice? Also at this point you can learn a lot from starting to practice basic push hands because push hands will illuminate your understanding of where you are in your practice. Of course there are two types of push hands, the first are the physical martial arts type where you see people basic wrestling trying to push off the other opponent until they realize the need to and become more refined. The second type of push hands, incorporate the Taiji principles and you learn what is missing in your forms practice. At this point you are practicing how to do push hands, learning how to yield to incoming force from an opponent and how the 13 energies work beginning with Peng, Lu, Ji, An. You may laugh at this point because if you do not have Peng you are quite aware where you are in your practice but that should not stop you. Remember everything you learn or become aware of becomes feedback to enhance, and improve your practice. Remember push hands just like weapons practice is a tool used to improve your skills and practice. Focus and be mindful of incorporating at this stage the following criteria: flexibility, relaxed energy (Song), central equilibrium, completeness, speed and quality. As you practice push hands begin to develop the listening skill called ting jin and neutralizing skills.

(3) Advanced

Advanced is the next level and you have now progressed and should be comfortable with the postures, and the classic principles. In order to get to the advanced level one must be aware of the principles of Taiji and now moving toward perfecting your internal practice. This requires more internal understanding and the heart/mind should be leading, your practice should be mindful of its internal organization and how it is operating. This is again a time to correct mistakes, hone skills, become much more smooth in your movement and more focused on your intent. The mind intent is now leading the Qi and the body is following. You are relaxing more and you are rooted. You have developed peng jin and understanding zhong ding (central equilibrium). At this point you are connected to the heaven and earth and you now understand yourself and beginning to understand fully your opponent.

When you practice you are not focused on the form or the Qi. You are now focusing on the flow, the stillness within movement, or the shen. Now you are doing your push hands and know how to do them, and are correcting your ability as you focus on utilizing the thirteen energies in your practice. You now can relax and let the true Taiji come out as you practice more internally. You now are centered and clear on what to do and how to practice to the point you feel you are definitely inside the door of Taiji and you have somewhat accomplished the ability to become a true Taiji practitioner. You are ready to move to the next level by observing what is happening internally and externally. You understand what it means to know yourself and your opponent and you fully realize Taiji is an internal art and all you need to do at this point is practice and persevere. You now are learning more about the function and applications of this internal martial art and how it positively affects your health and your martial arts skills. You love the art of Taiji and realize this great treasure. When you practice you are at peace and can emulate the classic principles, which you have studied and are now seeking to move on to practice the art of Taiji. You understand the phrase, "Best to be like water" (Laozi). You now know how to discharge energy and utilize it for self-defense. You want to continue on and deepen your practice. Your movements and Qi now flow and your internal force is increasing. Focus and mindfulness should now be how one reacts in their natural environment, how one incorporates the five elements, their root, the ability to neutralize and issue power and the ability to not rely on strength or LI. This includes the ability to practice and begin to excel at push hands.

(4) Mastery

You now understand yourself and are relaxed, enjoying your practice and feel free to focus on what you feel you need to and are observing any corrections you feel you need to make. The internal force is flowing and circulating throughout your body system. You practice differently then the students still learning to sense internal flow nuisances. You have practiced and persevered and mastery is now here and you have cultivated Dong jin. You now understand the life practice of many masters who practice, teach others, support this art and practice the art of Taiji as an art for art sake. What this means is you know how to defend yourself, and you are healthier and now you seek the higher ideals not just for fighting. New levels are pulling you up the mountain of inner attainment. You are not looking to fight mindlessly or just doing exercise for health but you want to know about the miraculous and what else is there on top of the mountain.

You have seen the light and this now is a more spiritual practice and you are following your heart because you love this art. You want to spread the word, help those trying to climb, share your knowledge, be happy and at peace. You have or are obtaining and now understand the difference between cultivating health, self-defense as a martial art, and art as a martial art. You have become Taiji and are one with the Universe and want to practice this universal art with all who love this art as you do. So you continue to refine and learn from your own practice and the practice of others by teaching them this great treasure called the art of Taiji. You understand the phrase, "Draw him in to land on nothing with four ounces moving a thousand pounds." (Laozi)

Insight

We mention four ounces moving a thousand pounds but it literally means that we use a small amount of effort to move a large amount of effort. We may use four ounces to move 500 pounds or a thousand but the importance that we reserve our energy and strength and only use a small amount to move all of our opponent's strength. At the same time we only allow the opponent to place 4 ounces on us, and not his thousand pounds of strength. We now understand we are cultivating ourselves on many levels because our consciousness has changed or is changing. Some who previously focused on fighting or only self-defense need to change their consciousness and focus less about learning Taijiquan for fighting and more about the Higher level art.

Master Chen Xaiowang

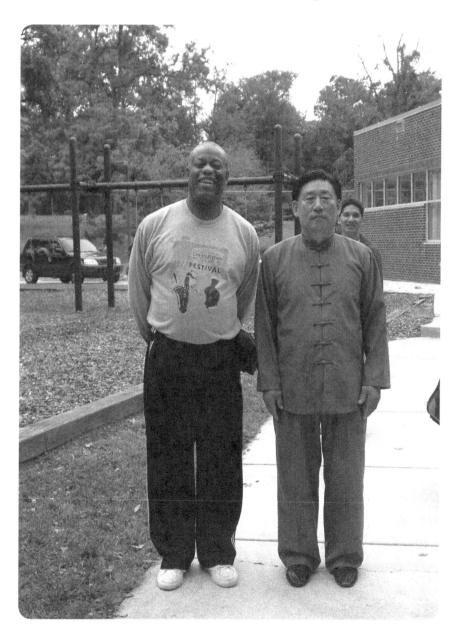

Chen Master Wang ZhenHua with Author in China

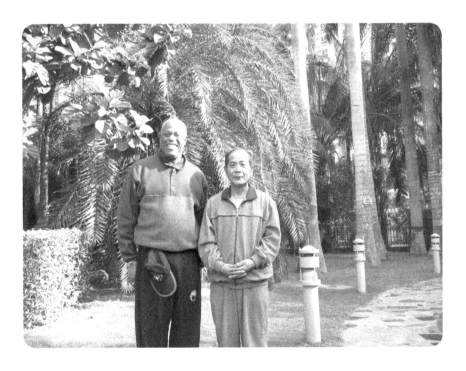

QI Rising
By George Samuels

QI rising isn't surprising
As the smoke clears
I wonder where the Qi went
As I clear my mind
Intent on being centered
To distinguish what is left of me
Or to my right

As I turn to meet the incoming
I don't duck
Instead I relax
The Sun shines
As we absorb its energy
Qi moves toward me
I await to feel its rays

Then I absorb all it has to deliver
Down to the ground
I realize it is time
To give back
To the one who has delivered it
As they await my next move
I turn to a new day

In a new way
They can't distinguish
Their right or left
And I push them off
Only for them to try
And turn away
But the force is moving too fast

As this is the case
When you turn first

They try to escape
Only to be locked
And now realize there is no place to go
But I save them the embarrassment
And let them up to save face
So we start again
This time I will wait
For their next move
Like the child waits on the dinner plate
Calm and anxious
Because I know it will be good

As they move
I move first
Sensing their energy
As they are late
I sink then turn them
as they lose balance and slip
And can't get away
But we laugh
To stop and yet await
To play another day.

IV

THE ART
(Ling Kong Jing)

Art of Chinese Calligraphy

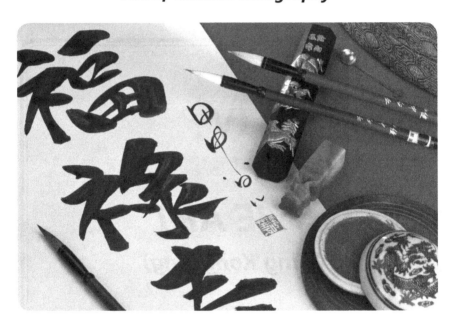

The Art

The art of Taijiquan is something that is not discussed amongst neophytes who want to become masters because Taiji like other internal martial arts in the past were considered to be transmitted from family to family, village to village and discussions of the higher levels were mostly discussed amongst masters or certain disciples of the art. These skills were imperative to protect family, food, money and lives. Now Taiji has grown beyond its borders and has spread to the world.

Most of the time Masters of the art feel most people would not understand so it would be a waste of time to discuss the art or highest levels unless one has proven they have the demonstrated higher level skills and have an understanding of the art on their level. This is the same as discussing black box technology with sport jocks who only know baseball or basketball. But this conversation will eventually have to be articulated with practitioners, new teachers and all masters reaching a high level of practicing Taiji. They should eventually be practicing for art sake. When I was in China I met a group of very high level Masters who were gracious enough to show me a few of their skills. They all were internal masters from different styles and at their level the style didn't matter. They explained that the principles were paramount. When I questioned their high level skills and how they got to that level they all stated that they practiced Taiji and other internal martial arts such as Taiji, Baqua, Xingyi, and He Liu Ba Fa as an art. They explained that they were artists (experts) and they had mastered the art. It's like cars; there are innumerable styles and models but they all will get you from home to the store and back home again. The overriding skill is can you drive. If you have the skill you can drive any car. Some drive a mustang, jeep, while some drive a Bentley, Roll Royce or Jaguar. The best drivers race cars, which, requires a high level of skills. It's the same in Taiji or internal martial arts. This inspired me to pursue the high art of Taiji and internal martial and healing arts.

This high art is different than any basic physical combat skills. It can become a life's work, which some consider to be now on a spiritual level where one is only concerned about the art and not the fighting. If you have not met those who focus only on the art level you may in the future and you will at least understand what they are focusing on and not just about fighting and who can best the other. One practices winning for win's sake, one on another level practices art for art's sake. Think about it for future thought.

What does the word "art," mean?

According to Wikipedia **Art** is a diverse range of human activities and the products of those activities which focuses primarily on the visual arts

According to Bing Dictionary meaning of **art** is:

- creation of beautiful things: the creation of beautiful or thought-provoking works, e.g. in painting, music, or writing
- beautiful objects: beautiful or thought-provoking works produced through creative activity
- branch of art: a branch or category of art, especially one of the visual arts

Art can be also identified as a work of art in dancing, performances such as competitions and would include martial arts such as Taiji. Art assumes a high level of skill beyond the mediocre and a love of, dedication and an accomplishment of a goal.

Again what is art?

Art is the pinnacle of practicing an art for arts' sake (艺至上主义yi zhi shang zhuyi). The art is connected to the art of nature, the love, the shen, and the spiritual nature of the universe. Taijiquan is an art and is connected to the spiritual universal and to Nature. From Wuji to yin yang then back to Wuji, full circle. The importance within the art is to use the art for healing oneself, self-cultivation, later others and refining ones' spirit for wisdom and developing inner peace. Art is being in harmony with others, the universe and us.

Insight: when is art not art (艺术yishu)?

Art is not art when you think that you are doing the art just for health or just as a physical martial art used for fighting only. Not realizing it is so much more, that is why it is called grand ultimate fist. When one practices the forms only they may or may not have any real function. Some masters describe internal martial art from the aspect of "skill", "technique", "art', "achievement" and the "Dao". This is why internal martial arts like Taijiquan are considered an art.

The Art of Function

Form versus function

There are different concepts of form and function such as:

- form for health to improve function,
- form for professional art,
- function for combat no art,
- function for combat with art,
- function for art with no fighting
- function for cultivation of consciousness

What is more important form or function? Once one learns forms from any particular style one must move to the next level and that is called function. Many people know a lot of forms, styles and can perform them well but few can perform the function. Many times forms are taught separate from function, which is a mistake liken to baking a pie with only the shell and no filling. Some may say it is best to first learn the form then add the function. This may be correct if you don't add any bad habits while learning the form. Once learning the form if one wants to move higher or deeper in their practice one must eventually learn function. Many times function is not taught because it takes longer to teach function and it takes time, practice and perseverance to learn and understand function. To incorporate function one must have a teacher who understands and have mastered function and/or can teach how one functions as an internal Taiji practitioner in order to master it. It may sound simplistic but it is not and it will require understanding how each posture functions and how you are supposed to function within the art of Taijiquan.

Function will make the difference between a Taiji practitioner and a Taiji master. When one learns how to perform external martial arts one is taught how to function because one is exposed to his or her external environment. When one who is an internal martial artist learning to function requires one to look inside at the same time as they are dealing in a similar external environment. The inside must function not just the external. This is where many get confused and perform external functions without learning or teaching the inside function. One has to be mindful of themselves first then the opponent. First one has to know them self inside then out. For example, one must be fully aware of yin and yang, substantial and insubstantial, and rooting along with central equilibrium. There are much more one needs to be aware of such as Song but it goes deeper because one must also be aware of the same criteria within the opponent. One must also be able to perform everything in unison, this is a requirement for mastery of Taijiquan.

Once you learn how to function inside then you will know how the opponent functions and how to apply that functionality to the opponent such as deflecting a thousand pounds using 4 ounces of strength. Many teachers and masters will train functionality once you have learned, practiced the postures and have a good foundation including an understanding of the basics. Learning functionality is just as important as learning push hands. You ask why, and the answer is that it will help your form to be better and more correct. It will improve your practice and help to correct mistakes one makes when they are unaware of how certain things such as push hands, applications and how to apply techniques you have learned. This is different than a great picture or winning a medal at a competition. Do you know what is more important; yin and yang or central equilibrium? They are both vital and of major importance. If you cannot function you will realize it when you practice push hands. Push hands will assist you with the knowledge of what is functioning in your forms and what is not. So it will help you to learn how the forms function, correct and improve your functioning.

Insight

All of that training and practice for those who will become masters of the art must learn how the art of Taiji functions within and beyond the forms. Everyone can learn to drive a car but few can drive it in the Grand Prix race of champions. It is not the same as driving down the street. Just the same as many can learn the forms and can win many medals but when confronted in a fight one may not be able to utilize what they have learned, how to function to protect themselves. Once a friend was attacked but had not practiced or understood the function of the postures and instead of utilizing his trained skills he froze and panicked. Later when I explained the functions of the forms he then realized he knew what to do if he had practiced the functions of the postures.

So forms are important to learn and practice, and for learning how this great art of Taijiquan functions in order to master and practice the art. One additional importance, understanding the classics will assist you with understanding the function of Taiji and its forms, energies, and intricacies. Additional information left by masters must be studied and absorbed such as the "Song of Substance and Function" so we too can function at a high level.

Song of Substance and Function

1. Taijiquan. Thirteen postures. The marvel lies in the nature of Qi; yin and yang.
2. It changes into infinity and returns to the one, Taijiquan.
3. The two primary principles (yin and yang) and four manifestations are without boundary.
   To ride the wind, the head is suspended at the crown, from above.
4. I have words for those who can understand: "If the yonquan (bubbling well) has no root, or the yao (waist) has no control, life long practice will be in vain".
5. There is no secret about the substance and function, they interrelate. The only way is to let wide and flowing Qi extend into the fingers.
6. Always remain in central equilibrium during peng (ward off), lu (roll-back), ji (press), an (push), cai (pluck), lie (split), zhou (elbow strike) and kao (lean-on), and also when steeping forward, sitting backward, looking left, looking right, and staying centered.
7. Neutralizing without neutralizing, yielding without yielding. Sit back before you move forward.
8. When the body is like a cloud, the whole body functions as the hands. The hands are not [only] the hands.
9. The mind must always remain aware.

(Reference: The Song of Substance translated by Wee Kee Jin Taijiquan Wuwei: A Natural Process ISBN 9780473097813)

Insight

This treatise above is the way of understanding the importance of function within your practice of Taiji. So that one will have substance inside of their forms and postures that demonstrate function after practicing for a long time since many practitioners have practiced for 10 or 20 years without any substance and function within their forms. Which is normal but by following the classic principles one has gained substance and function from properly practicing correctly. There is an old saying that states; if one practices for a long time one should be like a bag filled with substances that make the bag feel heavy. When opened the bag reveal all kinds of things learned, skills mastered and other stuff inside of it. On the otherhand If the the bag is opened and there is only a puff of air then one has not gained the substance of the art but just the hot air.

This will then lead one to the next level of being successful at pushing hands and applications. If the inside of you is functioning properly then you will have gained the substance and the skill of dong jin and appreciate the higher art of Taijiquan. The classics lead the way.

Grandmaster YunYinSen Liuhebafa ball training

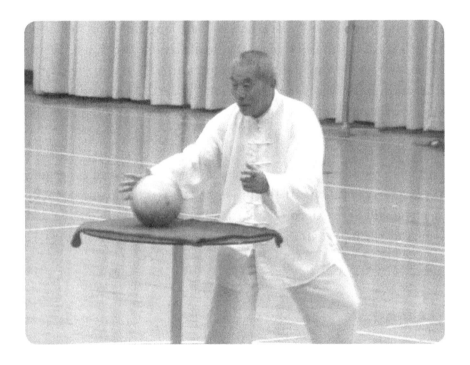

Grandmaster YunYinSen at Internal Martial Arts Camp in China 2007

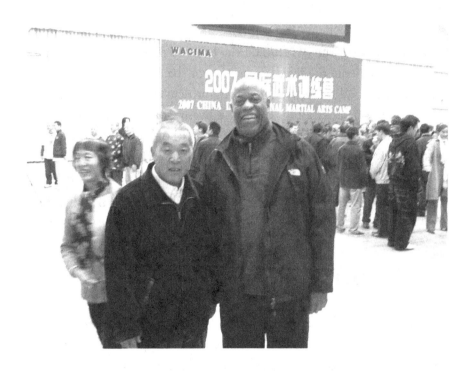

Back to the Classics, Excerpts of Taijiquan Classics states,

"From extreme softness one can then attain extreme hardness."
Externally, practice to train the tendons, bones, and skin; internally, practice to train the breath." Ancient practitioners of Daoism understood that in sitting meditation it is better to breathe in a way that is deep, tranquil, slow, and soft. Therefore, Lao Tzu, in his DaodeJing (道德经(Tao Te Ching), said, "Can we concentrate the mind to breathe softly like a child?"

In summary, after one has trained the body to perform slow, soft, and circular movements modeled after those of the sun, moon, earth, and other celestial bodies, with the guiding principles of circle after circle, circling connecting circling, cycling movements that are continuous, without excess, deficiency, or hollows, and without any abrupt stopping or sudden chopping, with the upper and lower parts of the body following each other, with yin and yang constantly interchanging, and with breathing that is even, soft, deep, tranquil, and long—then one can easily judge what the real Taijiquan is.

Insight of Taiji Structure

Taiji uses the mind intent and foundational structure so that one can use gravity and leverage to uproot and pull their opponents off balance. This is done through staying centered, turning the waist and using the legs to deliver the necessary energy to uproot the opponent. A level can move a thousand pound rock but one cannot pick it up with their hands. In order to move a heavy force directed at you, you must be able to turn or use leverage to divert the weight and force away from you. This is called the fulcrum point, which is the point at which one can dislodge a rock or lift a car with a jack.

This is why the art of Taiji is considered to be like a ball that can yield no matter how hard you hit it or apply force to it and the ball will return the same force back to the opponent. So when you practice you are trying to reach a place where your structure can duplicate the ball and be able to absorb and return the opponents force using leverage and the fulcrum points to uproot them utilizing the Taiji basic postures you have learned.

It is important to know that Taiji has an outer and inner structure and that the inner structure is the imperative because Taiji is internal. One must learn and practice the inner internal and focus on it just like a fisherman focuses on the fish inside the water and not on the water the boat sits on.

The fisherman places the fishing rod and hook in the water with a rod that is flexible and sensitive to anything touching the hook. This is similar to ting jin listening skill. The tip of the rod yields and is very flexible liken to the tip of a bamboo tree. Like the bamboo tree when touched it will give and bend until it reaches its maximum springy point and then will spring back whatever force is applied to it plus power. Nature has a way of demonstrating Taiji principles within so we can see clearly how they are applied and can draw an inference to our practice of Taijiquan.

This is the way to mastery of internal martial arts. Since Taiji is an internal art and one must insure that the internal gong is part of the practice and the main focus as opposed to the outer structure of the forms. Both are required but like the chicken and the egg. The eggs come from inside the chicken to the outside. Also the internal practice leads to the advanced skills and techniques of the art of Taiji. The classics again help us to understand all of this.

The Treatise On T'aiji Q'uan 王宗岳Wang Zongyue

太极者，无极而生，动静之机，阴阳之母也。动之则分，静之则合。无过不及，随曲就伸。人刚我柔谓之'走'，我顺人背谓之'粘'。动急则急应，动缓则缓随。虽变化万端，而理唯一贯。由着熟而渐悟懂劲，由懂劲而阶及神明。然非用力之久，不能豁然贯通焉！

虚领顶劲，气沉丹田，不偏不倚，忽隐忽现。左重则左虚，右重则右杳。仰之则弥高，俯之则愈深。进之则愈长，退之则愈促。一羽不能加，蝇虫不能落。人不知我，我独知人。英雄所向无敌，盖皆由此而及也！

斯技旁门甚多，虽势有区别，概不外壮欺弱、快欺慢耳！有力打无力，手慢让手快，是皆先天自然之能，非关学力而有为也！察'四两拨千斤'之句，显非力胜；观耄[mào]　耋[dié]能御众之形，快何能为？

立如平准，活似车轮。偏沉则随，双重则滞。每见数年纯功，不能运化者，率皆自为人制，双重之病未悟耳！

欲避此病，须知阴阳；粘即是走，走即是粘；阴不离阳，阳不离阴；阴阳相济，方为懂劲。懂劲后愈练愈精，默识揣摩，渐至从心所欲。

本是'舍己从人'，多误'舍近求远'。所谓'差之毫厘，谬之千里'，学者不可不详辨焉！是为论

The Treatise On T'aiji Q'uan 王宗岳Wang Zongyue

(Attributed to [Wang Zongyue] (18th Century) English translation

Taiji [Supreme Ultimate] comes from Wuji [Formless Void] and is the mother of yin and yang. In motion Taiji separates; in stillness yin and yang fuse and return to Wuji. It is not excessive or deficient; it follows a bending, adheres to an extension.

When the opponent is hard and I am soft, it is called tsou [yielding]. When I follow the opponent and he becomes backed up, it is called nian [adhering/sticking].

If the opponent's movement is quick, then quickly respond; if his movement is slow, then follow slowly.

Although there are innumerable variations, the principle that pervades them remains the same.

From familiarity with the correct touch, one gradually comprehends Jin [intrinsic strength]; from the comprehension of Jin one can reach wisdom.

Without long practice one cannot suddenly understand Taiji. Effortlessly the Jin reaches the top of the head. Let the Qi [vital life energy] sink to the dan-tien [field of elixir].

Don't lean in any direction; suddenly appear, suddenly disappear.

Empty the left wherever a pressure appears, and similarly the right.

If the opponent rises up, I seem taller; if he sinks down, then I seem lower; advancing, he finds the distance seems incredibly long; retreating, the distance seems exasperatingly short.

A feather cannot be placed, and a fly cannot alight on any part of the body. The opponent does not know me; I alone know him.

To become a peerless boxer results from this.

There are many boxing arts internal and external. Although they use different forms, for the most part they don't go beyond the strong dominating the weak, and the slow resigning to the swift. The strong defeating the weak and the slow hands ceding to the swift hands are all the results of natural abilities and not of well-trained techniques. From the sentence "A force of four ounces deflects a thousand pounds" we know that the technique is not accomplished with strength. The spectacle of an old person defeating a group of young people, how can it be due to swiftness? Stand like a perfectly balanced scale and move like a turning wheel. Sinking to one side allows movement to flow; being double-weighted is sluggish. **Anyone who has spent years of practice and still cannot neutralize, and is always controlled by his opponent, has not apprehended the fault of double-weightedness.**

Insight

To avoid this fault one must distinguish yin from yang. To adhere means to yield. To yield means to adhere. Within yin there is yang. Within yang there is yin. Yin and yang mutually aid and change each other. Understanding this you can say you understand Jin. After you understand Jin, the more you practice, the more skill.

Silently treasure knowledge and turn it over in the mind. Gradually you can do as you like. Fundamentally, it is giving up yourself to follow others. Most people mistakenly give up the near to seek the far. It is said, "Missing it by a little will lead many miles astray." The practitioner must carefully study. *Cheng Man Ching said, give a little, gain a little, and give a lot gain a lot.* This is vital because many try but do not succeed because the fault of double weightedness can be difficult to understand. The answer is in yin and yang, substantial and insubstantial so if you understand these terms and can demonstrate this in your form you will be able to demonstrate this in push hands. Double weightedness also includes understanding force, not just the weight only. You can make one leg substantial and the other insubstantial but you must understand that force in one leg means no force in the other leg. If you have one arm substantial the other is insubstantial. This can be interpreted as yin and yang. This means that yin and yang is everywhere and when you meet the opponent's yang force against you, it requires you to become yin otherwise it will be force against force. Then you will avoid the fault of double weightedness.

Practicing Pushing (Sensing) Hands

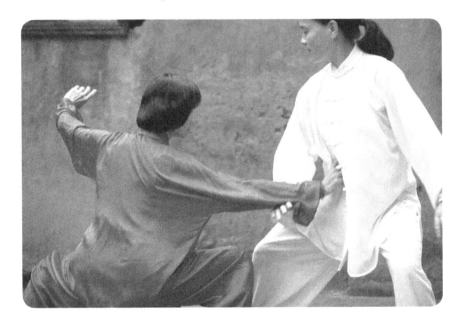

Go Ahead Push
By George Samuels

Go ahead and push
I see you
You can't see me
I am in front of you
Now I am behind you
You attack
I disappear
Then reappear
Only to step
Into your space
You don't know what to do
I cover you
As I capture your center
Imbalanced to try to run
But I run faster
You withdraw I send you flying
You land only to try and take off again
I am there before you
As we laugh
And practice yet again

The Art of Push Hands

Sensing hands or Push hands

You touch me, I touch you so what? What does it mean unless I can sense your internals, your energy, your tension, your bone, your speed, your yin or yang or li (muscle strength). What am I using to do all of this analysis? My senses, which are all of them and this includes my hand. When I touch you I am sensing, not just touching for no reason. My hands are for sensing, what are your hands for? Are sensitive enough so you can feel a feather touch you anywhere? Are you so sensitive you can feel a fly alight or a bird cannot push off from your sensitivity and ability to yield its futile efforts? Do you know your opponent but he does not know you? Can you give to receive?

Loss and Gain

In push hands one has to learn to give up to get, give to receive and invest in loss to win. Cheng Man Ching stated this and many other Masters so one will understand the difference between force against force, and yielding to the incoming force. Taiji is an internal practice and not an external practice that seems to reveal itself when some begin to do push hands and resort to wrestling. This again causes us to go back to the classics to fully understand what to do, or research, or listen to our Teacher. How do we correct our misunderstandings or mistakes. Cheng Man Ching stated; give a little, gain a little, give up a big loss to gain a big win. His statement and the importance of understanding of the art of Taiji teaches us to utilize our minds and skills in order to win by utilizing the wisdom of Taiji and not settle for the small immediate gain and later on suffering a big loss. This is all about skills and understanding how to function as a Taiji Master when confronted by any situation. Practice does make perfect especially when we follow the masters who gave us the information and knowledge of how to accomplish these high level skills such as Peng, Lu, JI and An.

Song of Push Hands （打手歌dashouge）

掤捋挤按须认直，上下相随人难进。

任他巨力来打我，牵动四两拨千斤。

引进落空合即出，沾连黏随不丢顶。

Be conscientious in Peng, Lu, Ji, and An.

SONG OF PUSH HANDS

(by Unknown Author as researched by Lee N. ScheeleEnglish translation)

Be conscientious in Peng, Lu, Ji, and An.

Upper and lower coordinate, and the opponent finds it difficult to penetrate.

Let the opponent attacks with great force; use four ounces to deflect a thousand pounds.

Attract to emptiness and discharge; zhan (touch), Lian (connect), nian (stick), Sui (follow), attach without losing the attachment.

Insight

One can master the forms but the next step is the function of the postures and then exhibiting that ability within push hands practice. Theory is fine but one must be able to demonstrate they have put it into practice. Then you must train to show what you have learned and your progress as you continue your practice. We may think we have it all in mind but the body must also be able to demonstrate that all is working seamlessly together as one unit in unison. This is where form meets function. This is where disharmony meets harmony.

My Teacher Grandmaster Lui Bao Yu and his disciple Master Lilly Gao in China practicing push hands

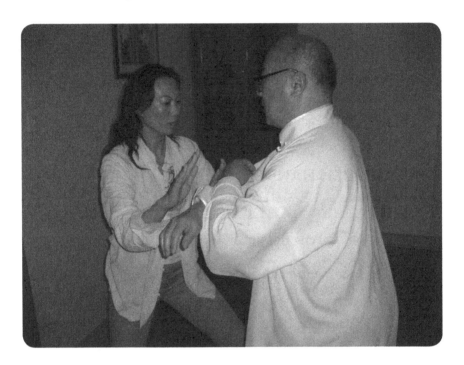

When is a hand not a hand?

When you are the hand and the hand then is not a hand. Should I hit your head to make you understand this most important point? Think about it when you are practicing push hands.

When doing push hands, what are some of the most important factors especially when an opponent is attacking us?

- Listen
- Give up and follow
- Stickiness
- Determine distance

- Determine space
- Determine force
- Measure timing
- Neutralize
- Follow until we can take advantage after leading the opponent into a disadvantaged position
- Lead them into emptiness
- Absorb and project
- Empty and full
- Protect, defend and attack and at the right time
- Remember the 5 bows and becoming one big bow
- Central equilibrium

The Philosophy of Folding

Another additional skill one must understand and practice is the art of folding. When one practices the art of push hands and Da Lu one must understand how to do folding. Folding is accomplished when the opponent grabs your hand that you fold and use your elbow. When the opponent locks your arm you use your shoulder. When the opponent locks your arm and shoulder you use your body. When the opponent restricts or locks your body you use your foot. Understanding this will also apply to using the 13 energies starting with the four Peng, Lu Ji An. Once an opponent touches your body you apply the techniques of stick, connect, adhere and follow and use folding to defend yourself.

Insight

This idea and principles of pushing hands or sensing hands or pushing body is required to understand so one can succeed at pushing hands. Once the confusion of what you are supposed to know is cleared up and what you are supposed to understand perfectly is clear, then you will equally understand terms and contradiction of terms. The importance is to understand hands are not hands and touching the opponent is not for touching but for sensing. One should develop listening skill called ting jin （听劲）. Listening and sensing go hand in hand and once perfected serves as our ability to know our opponents while they know us. Listening and sensing skills will help you to be able to know when the opponent moves so you can move first and neutralize the opponent's incoming force. It will also help you to locate the opponents' center.

Once understood and clear one can move to a level of excelling at push hands and how to utilize your neutralization skills (Dong jin) of Taiji for martial arts applications. Again review and study the classics to insure you have incorporated all of the vital techniques and you understand the different thirteen energies. One other benefit of practicing push hands will help you to remove the rough edges on the (your) ball until it is smooth. First you learn to neutralize then you learn how to push, attack (fajin) and then use more advanced techniques. Then we reach the level of being able to neutralize and attack at the same time. We will be able harmonize our inner and outer self.

Combat and Self-defense

For combat one must remember to train for combat which require practicing the basic drills used in the fighting arts such as Muay Tai, or Boxing, or Wing Chun or Shaolin gongfu or Kick boxing. This means one must train punching, blocking, kicking, learn how to attack, and to protect and understand the strategy of combat. Also one should practice two-man forms. There are many schools of combat theory from external gongfu to internal arts such as Taiji and Xingyi and Bagua. Different strategies comprise some of these examples:

- there is the idea of stick and adhere then follow the opponent closely and strike directly

- move forward and attack until opponent is finished
- circle, move and deflect until one finds a weak point
- wait until one is attacked then defend
- sneak attack at the first sign of trouble

There are a multitude of strategies but the overall objective is to defend oneself and win the battle. I say there is one technique that outweighs them all which is:

- do not get in a fight,
- avoid a fight if you see one coming
- do not instigate a fight
- winning is not the answer, not fighting is
- sometimes in a fight there is no winner or loser

You might think you know the answer but many times the winner of fights is not the one who walks away with less bruises. I say live to fight another day. Sometimes the winner is the one who avoided the fight or did not fight at all because they used wisdom.

Wisdom comes from survivors and peacemakers not warriors but one must be prepared to defend oneself in case they cannot just walk away from a fight and it is inevidentable. I have avoided many fights by using wisdom even when I knew I would win. But there have been times I could not avoid the fight so I had to defend and protect myself by any means necessary. When this happens then one must rely on

- Training,
- Practice
- Skills and techniques
- Strategy

First and foremost one needs to get in shape and stay in shape through training. This is why it is important to practice forms, postures and basic gongfu techniques. For example punching the bag helps because if you never punched anything you will not win any fights especially if you cannot make a proper fist. Second practice simple basic skills using fist, hand, leg, knee, elbows is step one. How to use the basic weapons you have helps. How to block; punches, kicks, and etc. also helps. Thirdly learning simple techniques, developing application skills also helps especially when the opponent has their hands on you. Learning different techniques even simple one will help especially if the opponent is stronger or bigger than you or even tougher. Also when you practice you learn how to control fear, which is paramount, not that you are scare of the opponent but also you might be scare of getting hurt. So you must show guts or inner strength. Some high-level martial artists are scared they might hurt the opponent (smile), truth. Fourth you must have a strategy or two so that when you are in a troublesome situation you know how you are going to deal with the opponent(s). This is very important and it will save your life. *In Taiji there is no opposition, "If you do not compete…(Laozi)*

Ask yourself what should I do if I am in this type of situation or not do. For example, a friend of mine was on the way home, was approached by a robber with a gun. The gunman demanded their purse. She immediately slapped him with it. He turned and said, I can just shoot you instead of just taking your purse. She shocked realized she should just give up the purse that only had eight dollars in it. So she gave it to him and he left the scene. The slapping of the gunman with the purse only pissed him off, not the best idea. Another situation I was in when a guy and his friends tried to harass me by the leader of the gang of martial artists said I looked weak and out of shape. The leader came over with his crew and shoved me while the gang laughed. I smile as I sized up the gang members to see who was tough and who was not. Then the leader came over and told me I was weak and what could I do. Sensing he was up to no good I then realized there was no way out so I used his tough martial arts skills against him. I used my Taiji chansijin (Chen style) training by inviting him to try that again. He obliged me by trying to shove me again with both hands. I could see he was strong, he had lots of muscles with a bad attitude but when he tried to shove me I just rooted and turned as he almost fell to the ground but I did not use my hands so his friends would not jump in. I just then invited him again and again to try and shove me and he could not. Then I told him I could shove him all over and he could not stop me so he said ok try. Smiling I shoved him using yin yang all over the place until he realized he could not stop me. He then told his boys to try and the biggest guy came and tried and failed. Seeing that he looked bad and was losing face he then asked me what did I practice and I said Taiji. Realizing this he decided to invite me to join his group but I declined and instead said we could be friends, which he agreed. We all laughed and they went about their business and I mine. Now when I see them we just say Hi. The moral of the story is to understand to not look for fights but to use wisdom to avoid fights when you can. If you have to fight use your strategy and skills to defend yourself. This does not matter if it is external or internal martial arts.

As in Taijiquan we use different skills, techniques and strategies to defend ourselves. But as in combat the outcome is the same to avoid getting hurt and defending ourselves against aggression and attacks. So how do we do this in Taijiquan. We should use principles that we have learned such as:

- *Feeling*: sensing the opponents force, direction, speed, level of force, strength, weakness and attacking at that weak point
- *Neutralizing*: yielding to the oncoming attack, not using our force against the opponents force but changing the direction of that force using a circular strategy and leading that force into emptiness until it is neutralized
- *Controlling:* avoiding the opponent's main force, targeting their weak point(s), and putting ourselves into an advantageous position to attack
- *Attacking:* when we find the weak point(s) to attack until the opponent is immobilized and the attack is over

- *Excessive force:* using whatever force is necessary and then knowing when to stop if the opponent has given up or is immobilized, no need to finish the opponent to prove our skill. This is important because unnecessary force is not using wisdom. We protect and defend not go around attacking others to prove we are tough.

Being Taiji is an internal martial art one must focus not on the external. Our focus is on using our skill of interpreting the energy of the opponent. Using the internal skills we have developed, and the energies we have perfected such as ward off, rollback, push, elbow stroke and etc. we can lead the opponents energy into emptyness and then issuing force.

Song of Sparring

(from Lost Tai-chi Classics from the late Ching Dynasty by Douglas Wile)

> *Be serious in the practice of ward-off, roll-back, press and push*
> *And in pull-down, split, elbow-stroke, and shoulder-stroke mind your bending and extending*
> *In advance retreat, gaze-left, look-right, and equilibrium,*
> *You must stick, connect, adhere, and follow, distinguishing full and empty*
> *The hands and feet follow each other, and the waist and legs act in unison;*
> *Drawing the opponent in so that his energy lands on nothing is a marvelous technique*
> *Let him attack with great force,*
> *While I deflect a thousand pounds with four ounces.*

Insight

Remember softness can overcome hardness and softness can turn into hardness. Also, use circular skills against linear skills, such as Taiji uses circular skills whereas other martial arts use linear skills such as in karate or boxing. Another point is to always remain calm, relaxed (Fang Song), energy sunk and ready. (Calm will beat out panic most of the time.) Sensing so that when the opponent moves you arrive first. Do not forget to breathe naturally. Yes four ounces can move a thousand pounds you just need to know how! You do not have to fight to prove you can fight. Sometimes if there was no fight everyone won, no one lost. The winners are those who get to go home safe, sound and healthy. Running is a strategy and technique also if required. Fighting a gang is no fun except on TV.

Part of learning skills requires us to know and practice the main vital postures utilized in Taijiquan. In Taijiquan we utilize not only physical attributes but also energetic and mental and spiritual attributes. So we must understand fully the eight energies and the five directions, which add up to thirteen postures. As part of this there are the eight main energies and how to understand their internal skills. The Song of Eight Postures expands upon their apparent physical meanings to their energetic and higher-level meanings.

Songs of The Eight Postures

(Attributed to T'an Meng-hsienas researched by Lee N. Scheele)

The Song of Peng

What is the meaning of Peng energy? It is like the water supporting a moving boat. First sink the ch'i to the tan-t'ien, then hold the head as if suspended from above. The entire body is filled with spring like energy, opening and closing in a very quick moment. Even if the opponent uses a thousand pounds of force, he can be uprooted and made to float without difficulty.

The Song of Lu

What is the meaning of Lu energy? Entice the opponent toward you by allowing him to advance, lightly and nimbly follow his incoming force without disconnecting and without resisting. When his force reaches its farthest extent, it will naturally become empty. The opponent can then be let go or countered at will. Maintain your central equilibrium and your opponent cannot gain an advantage.

The Song of Qi

What is the meaning of Qi energy? There are two aspects to its functional use: The direct way is to go to meet the opponent and attach gently in one movement. The indirect way is to use the reaction force like the rebound of a ball bouncing off a wall, or a coin thrown on a drumhead, bouncing off with a ringing sound.

The Song of An

What is the meaning of An energy? When applied it is like flowing water. The substantial is concealed in the insubstantial. When the flow is swift it is difficult to resist. Coming to a high place, it swells and fills the place up; meeting a hollow it dives downward. The waves rise and fall, finding a hole they will surely surge in.

The Song of Tsai

What is the meaning of Ts'ai energy? It is like the weight attached to the beam of a balance scale. Give free play to the opponent's force no matter how heavy or light, you will know how heavy or light it is after weighing it. To push or pull requires only four ounces, one thousand pounds can also be balanced. If you ask what the principle is, the answer is the function of the lever.

The Song of Lie

What is the meaning of Lie energy? It revolves like a spinning disc. If something is thrown onto it, it will immediately be cast more than ten feet away. Have you not seen a whirlpool form in a swift flowing stream? The waves roll in spiraling currents. If a falling leaf drops into it, it will suddenly sink from sight.

The Song of Zhou

What is the meaning of Zhou energy? Its method relates to the Five Elements. Yin and Yang are divided above and below. Emptiness and substantiality must be clearly distinguished. Joined in unbroken continuity, the opponent cannot resist the posture. Its explosive pounding is especially fearsome. When one has mastered the six kinds of energy, the applications become unlimited.

The Song of K'ao

What is the meaning of K'ao energy? Its method is divided into the shoulder and back technique. In Diagonal Flying Posture use shoulder, but within the shoulder technique there is also some use of the back. Once you have the opportunity and can take advantage of the posture, the technique explodes like pounding a pestle. Carefully maintain your own center of gravity. Those who lose it will have no achievement.

Insight

As one grows in their practice one must understand the energies they are utilizing and how to manipulate them. One important thing to understand is that when one is learning and unfamiliar with much of what they are reading or researching it is best to seek an understanding from your teacher or any master so you understand and to clear up any confusion.

What is the most important energy out of the eight? The first four energies are important (Peng, Lu, Ji, and An.) The most important of these is Peng. If one has Peng then all else is possible. Once one has gained Peng one can become like the proverbial ball and utilize the Peng energy instead of bone or Li (physical strength). If you throw a rock at a ball it will bounce off with the springy type energy. This also confirms one's ability to root and connect to Earths' energy and that the energy is flowing throughout the body system. Then all the other energies can be mobilized. Without Peng one will have to use Li. Once you have mastered these energetic skills then you are ready to move on to learning higher-level skills. Practice using the energies within your fixed step push hands first then move on to moving step and free style until it becomes automatic. This is part of developing higher-level skills and it requires much to understand an art like Taijiquan. For example, there are additional requirements one must incorporate. The five-character secret helps to outline the process one should understand so read it over and over until it is clear.

清李亦畬太極拳論 (李亦畬)

Five Character Secret (tactics) by
Li I-yu {Qing Dynasty}

五字訣

一曰心靜：心不靜則不專，一舉手前後左右全無定向，故要心靜。起初舉動未能由己，要息心體認，隨人所動，隨屈就伸，不丟不頂，勿自伸縮。彼有力，我亦有力，我力在先；彼無力，我亦無力，我意仍在先。要刻刻留意，挨何處，心要用在何處，須向不丟不頂中討消息。從此做去，一年半載，便能施於身。此全是用意，不是用勁。久之，則人為我制，我不為人制矣！

二曰身靈：身滯則進退不能自如，故要身靈。舉手不可有呆像，彼之力方礙我皮毛，我之意已入彼骨內。兩手支撐，一氣貫串。左重則左虛，而右已去；右重則右虛，而左已去。氣如車輪，周身俱要相隨，有不相隨處，身便散亂，便不得力，其病於腰腿求之。先，以心使身，從人不從己；後，身能從心，由己仍是從人。由己則滯，從人則活。能從人，手上便有分寸，秤彼勁之大小，分釐不錯；權彼來之長短，毫髮無差。前進後退，處處恰合，功彌久而技彌精矣！

三曰氣斂：氣勢散漫，便無含蓄，身易散亂，務使氣斂入脊骨，呼吸通靈，周身罔間。吸為合、為蓄；呼為開、為發。蓋吸則自然提得起，亦拏得人起，呼則自然沉得下、亦放得人出。此是以意運氣，非以力使氣也！

四曰勁整：一身之勁，練成一家。分清虛實，發勁要有根源：勁起於腳根，主於腰間，形於手指，發於脊骨。又要提起全副精神，於彼勁將發未發之際，我勁已接入彼勁。恰好不先不後，如皮燃火，如泉湧出。前進後退，無絲毫散亂。曲中求直，蓄而後發，方能隨手奏效。此謂「借力打人」、「四兩撥千斤」也！

五曰神聚：上四者俱備，總歸神聚。神聚，則一氣鼓鑄，煉氣歸神，氣勢騰挪；精神貫注，開合有致，虛實清楚。左虛則右實，右虛則左實。虛，非全然無力，氣勢要有騰挪。實，非全然占煞，精神要貴貫注。緊要全在胸中、腰間變化，不在外面。力從人借，氣由脊發。胡能氣由脊發？氣向下沉，由兩肩收入脊骨，注於腰間，此氣之由上而下也，謂之「合」；由腰形於脊骨，布於兩膊，施於手指，此氣之由下而上也，謂之「開」。合便是收，開即是放。能懂開合，便知陰陽。到此地位，功用一日，技精一日，漸至從心所欲，罔不如意矣！

Five Character Secret

(by Li I-yu as researched by Lee N. Scheele) English translation

CALM

The hsin [mind-and-heart] should be calm. If the hsin is not calm, one cannot concentrate, and when the arm is raised, whether forward or back, left or right, it is completely without certain direction. Therefore, it is necessary to maintain a calm mind. The entire mind must also experience and comprehend the movements of the opponent. Accordingly, when the movement bends, it then straightens, without disconnecting or resisting. Do not extend or retreat by yourself. If my opponent has li [external strength], I also have li, but my li is previous in exact anticipation of his. If the opponent does not have li, I am also without li, but my Yi [mind-intent] is still previous. It is necessary to be continually mindful; to whatever part of the body is touched the mind should go. You must discover the information by non-discrimination and non-resistance. Follow this method, and in one year, or a half-year, you will instinctively find it in your body. All of this means you use I, not Jin [intrinsic force]. After practicing for a long time, the opponent will be controlled by me, and I will not be controlled by him.

AGILITY

If the body is clumsy, then in advancing or retreating it cannot be free; therefore, it must be agile. Once you raise your arm, you cannot appear clumsy. The moment the force of my opponent touches my skin and hair, my mind is already penetrating his bones. When holding up the arms, the Qi [vital life energy] is threaded together continuously. When the left side is heavy, it then empties, and the right side is already countering. When the right is heavy, it empties, and the left is already countering. The Qi is like a wheel, and the whole body must mutually coordinate. If there is any uncoordinated place, the body becomes disordered and weak. The defect is to be found in the waist and legs.

First the mind is used to order the body. Follow the opponent and not your own inclination. Later your body can follow your mind, and you can control yourself and still follow the opponent. When you only follow your own inclination, you are clumsy, but when you follow the opponent, then your hands can distinguish and weigh accurately the amount of his force, and measure the distance of his approach with no mistake. Advancing and retreating, everywhere the coordination is perfect. After studying for a long time, your technique will become skillful.

BREATH To Gather the Qi

If the Qi is dispersed, then it is not stored and is easy to scatter. Let the Qi penetrate the spine and the inhalation and exhalation be smooth and unimpeded throughout the entire body. The inhalation closes and gathers, the exhalation opens and discharges. Because the inhalation can naturally raise and also uproot the opponent, the exhalation can naturally sink down and also fa-jin [discharge energy] him. This is by means of the Yi, not the li mobilizing the Qi, which is standard for this style (Taiji).

INTERNAL FORCE The Complete Jin

The Jin of the whole body, through practice becomes one unit. Distinguish clearly between substantial and insubstantial. To fa-jin it is necessary to have root. The Jin starts from the foot, is commanded by the waist, and manifested in the fingers, and discharged through the spine and back. One must completely raise the shen [spirit of vitality] at the moment when the opponent's Jin is about to manifest, but has not yet been released. My Jin has then already met his, not late, not early. It is like using a leather (tinder) to start a fire, or like a fountain gushing forth. In going forward or stepping back, there is not even the slightest disorder. In the curve seek the straight, store, then discharge; then you are able to follow your hands and achieve a beautiful result. This is called borrowing force to strike the opponent or using four ounces to deflect a thousand pounds.

SPIRIT Shen Concentrated

Having the above four, then you can return to concentrated spirit: if the spirit is concentrated, then it is continuous and uninterrupted, and the practice of Qi returns to the shen [spirit of vitality]. The manifestation of Qi moves with agility. When the shen is concentrated, opening and closing occur appropriately, and the differentiation of substantial and insubstantial is clear. If the left is insubstantial, the right is substantial, and vice-versa. Insubstantial does not mean completely without strength. The manifestation of Qi must be agile. Substantial does not mean completely limited. The spirit must be completely concentrated. It is important to be completely in the mind (I) and the waist, and not outside. Not being outside or separated, force is borrowed from the opponent, and the Qi is released from the spine. How can the chi discharge from the spine? It sinks downward from the two shoulders, gathers to the spine, and pours to the waist. This is chi from up to down and is called closed. From the waist the Qi mobilizes to the spine, spreads to the two arms and flows to the fingers. This is Qi from down to up and is called opened. Closed is gathering, and opened is discharging. When you know opening and closing, then you know yin and yang. Reaching this level your skill will progress with the days and you can do as you wish.

Insight

The five-character secret is imperative to understand and to test to determine if you can deflect a thousand pounds with 4 ounces. If you can then you are in compliance, if you cannot then reread and see if you fully understand the function of your Taiji and push hands skills. See if you comply with what is written above. Practice more then ask yourself, am I able to perform the points above, if I cannot what do I need to understand, correct and/or practice. So study the classic treatises, which will provide the clues to what you are doing right or not doing. If you have a teacher then they will point out what you are doing correctly or what you need to do but if not the classic treatises can help you by giving more light on the essentials of the practice of the form and push-hands.

Yin Yang Symbol

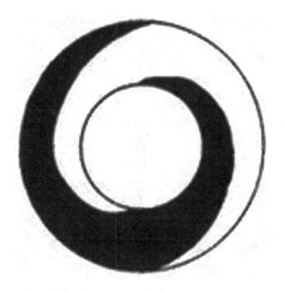

Essentials Of The Practice of The Form and Push-Hands

(by Li I-yu)

走架打手行工要言

　　昔人云:「能引進落空,能四兩撥千斤;不能引進落空,不能四兩撥千斤。」語甚概括。初學末由領悟,予加數語以解之。俾有志斯技者,得所從入,庶日進有功矣!

　　欲要引進落空,四兩撥千斤,先要知己知彼;欲要知己知彼,先要捨己從人;欲要捨己從人,先要得機得勢;欲要得機得勢,先要周身一家;欲要周身一家,先要周身無有缺陷;欲要周身無有缺陷,先要神氣鼓盪;欲要神氣鼓盪,先要提起精神,神不外散;欲要神不外散,先要神氣收斂入骨;欲要神氣收斂入骨,先要兩股前節有力,兩肩松開,氣向下沉。勁起於腳根,變換在腿,含蓄在胸,運動在兩肩,主宰在腰。上於兩膊相繫,下於兩胯、兩腿相隨。勁由內換,收便是合,放即是開。靜則俱靜。靜是合,合中寓開;動則俱動,動是開,開中寓合。觸之則旋轉自如,無不得力,才能引進落空,四兩撥千斤。

　　平日走架,是知己工夫。一動勢,先問自己:周身合上數項不合?少有不合,即速改換。走架所以要慢,不要快。打手,是知人工夫。動靜固是知人,仍是問己。自己要安排得好,人一挨我,我不動彼絲毫,趁勢而入,接定彼勁,彼自跌出。如自己有不得力處,便是雙重未化,要於陰陽開合中求之,所謂「知己知彼,百戰百勝」也!

　　胞弟啟軒嘗以毬譬之:如置毬於平坦,人莫可攀躋,強臨其上,向前用力——後跌,向後用力,前跌。譬喻甚明,細揣其理,非「捨己從人」、「一身一家」之明證乎?得此一譬,「引進落空」、「四兩撥千金」之理,可盡人而明矣!

Essentials Of The Practice of The Form and Push-Hands

(translation by Li I-yu)

Formerly people said: being able to attract to emptiness, you can use four ounces to deflect a thousand pounds, Not being able to attract to emptiness, you cannot deflect a thousand pounds. The words are simple, but the meaning is complete. The beginner cannot understand it. Here I add some words to explain it. If someone is ambitious to learn this art, he can find some way to enter it and every day he will have some improvement.

Desiring to attract to emptiness and deflect a thousand pounds, first you must know yourself and others. If you want to know yourself and others, you must give up yourself and follow others. If you give up yourself and follow others, first you must have the correct timing and position. To obtain the correct timing and position, you must first make your body one unit. Desiring to make the body one unit, you must first eliminate hollows and protuberances. To make the whole body without breaks or holes, you must first have the shen [spirit of vitality] and chi [vital life energy] excited and expanded. If you want the shen and chi activated and expanded, you must first raise the spirit (pay attention) and the shen should not be unfocussed. To have your shen not unfocussed, you must first have the shen and Qi gather and penetrate the bones. Desiring the shen and Qi to penetrate the bones, first you must strengthen the two thighs and loosen the two shoulders and let the Qi sink down.

The Jin [intrinsic strength] raises from the feet, changes in the legs, is stored in the chest, moved in the shoulders and commanded in the waist. The upper part connects to the two arms and the lower part follows the legs. It changes inside. To gather is to close and to release is to open. If it is quiet, it is completely still. Being still means to close. In closing there is opening. If it is moving, everything moves. Moving is open. In opening there is closing. When the body is touched it revolves freely. There is nowhere that does not obtain power. Then you can attract to emptiness and use four ounces to deflect a thousand pounds.

Practicing the Form every day is the gongfu of knowing yourself. When you start to practice, first ask yourself, "Did my whole body follow the above principles or not?" If one little place did not follow them, then correct it immediately. Therefore, in practicing the Form we want slowness not speed.

Push hands is the gongfu of knowing others. As for movement and stillness, although it is to know others, you must still ask yourself. If you arrange yourself well, when others touch you, you do not move a hair. Follow the opportunity and meet his Jin and let him fall naturally outward. If you feel someplace in your body is powerless, it is double-weighted and unchanging. You must seek the defect in yin and yang, opening and closing. Know yourself and know others: in one hundred battles you will win one hundred

Insight

The key points above will change your practice if we are lacking in some area. Part of our problem is to be aware of how we are progressing, what is missing and how to correct and do it correctly. If you practice and you are not improving look to the form and function, or your practice and do additional research of the classics. If you have a teacher ask for assistance. Then try to continue to practicing and researching. The steps to transferring power will further enlighten you.

The sixteen steps of transferring power

(Reference: Tai Chi Classics by Waysun Liao; ISBN 1570627495 p. 83)

1. *Root and twist the foot, allowing power to travel up the leg.*
2. *Let the power spring upward at the knee.*
3. *Allow the power to move freely in any direction at the waist.*
4. *Drive the power upward through the back.*
5. *Let the power penetrate to the crown point at the top of the head.*
6. *From the crown point, mingle the power with your Qi and circulate it through the entire body.*
7. *Drive the power to the palm.*
8. *Push the power to the fingertips.*
9. *Condense the power into the bone marrow throughout the entire body.*
10. *Merge the power with the spirit, making them one.*
11. *Listen with your mind at the ear, almost as if condensing slightly.*
12. *Concentrate at the area of your nose.*
13. *Breathe to the lungs.*
14. *Control the mouth, carefully regulating the breathing.*
15. *Spread the power to the entire body.*
16. *Push the power to the ends of body hairs.*

Insight

The essentials of the practice of the form and push-hands is teaching you the process that you must follow in order to be able to excel at push hands and how to use the practice of the forms to improve function. These words are not to be overlooked and were created so one will really understand how to practice step by step and what is to be gained. The sixteen steps are important because they provide the path the Jin will follow and understand how it will expand into the eight directions. The Jin travels throughout the body in order for one to use it for health and to strike with relaxed force..

Advanced Qi Skills

Once practitioners have achieved a level of success and mastery with push hands and fully understand their structure they want to be able to develop more higher internals skills. The classics help by explaining knowledge that one must know in order to progress and understand how to do from a purely internal perspective. For example the *"Four Word Secret Formula"* listed below.

Four Word Secret Formula By Wu Yu Xiang(Translation taken from T.Y. Pang's book, "On Tai Chi Chaun")

- ✓ To **Spread** is to circulate the Qi in my body, to spread it upon his strength so he cannot move freely.
- ✓ To **Cover** is to use my Qi to cover the point of his attack.
- ✓ To **Confront** is to use my Qi to match his approach precisely.
- ✓ To **Swallow** is to use my Qi to receive and transform his power completely.

Insightful Importance

These four words are formless and soundless. Only one who understands internal strength and achieves the finest stages can know the meaning of what has been said here about Qi. Only one who cultivates his Qi correctly so that it spreads to the body's four limbs will be able to respond to the soundlessness and formlessness of these four words. This is advanced and requires one to be able to use the qigong in a three to four dimensional way and beyond where the qi can go through everywhere and move from their intent. The consciousness is transformed and is functioning at a higher level as one continues to cultivate a higher understanding of higher-level martial arts.

More Personal Insights on Cultivating Higher Skills

There a multitude of higher skills that are cultivated as our consciousness and skills become more refined. Before moving forward one should be able to have mastered all the basic techniques otherwise one needs to go back and correct anything that is missing or incorrect. At this point you should be clear on all the points below:

Are you Alive?

Yes, then make sure you are alive within your practice. One of the things to recognize is that the masters of internal martial arts are alive. Taiji is alive and one is alive inside so ask yourself are you alive if not wake up, be alive. When one reaches a higher level and understands Taiji they must be alive inside. Taiji is live art not a dead art. It lives, moves and breathes life. Energy is life always moving, changing, and going from yin to yang and to Wuji. So ask yourself are you alive inside, if you do not know find out.

Are you Breathing?

Where is your breath? Do you know? Have you checked to see if it is deep or shallow? This must be checked and understood that the more you relax the deeper your breath. So relax be mindful that your breath is deeper when you are practicing. If not relax breathe naturally and don't you're your breath. Remember breathing helps to heal the body, harmonize the mind and spirit.

Are you Rooted?

You should be able to root and are rooted standing or moving while you practice. if not relax even more. Adjust your structure so that you are straight and aligned with the earth and heaven. Don't ignore this point. Do your (Zhanzhuang) more. This is required standing still and even when you are moving you must relax and maintain your root. If you discover that you have no power or losing power when you or try to strike then you are segmented and not part of a unitary body effort. This is because you have no root. Also the upper body and lower body must work together otherwise it will diminish your power. You can tell you are rooted when the upper body is light and the lower body is heavy. When one learns to root, he has much greater control of his own balance as well as greater potential of power coming from the ground. Then one can use the lower body to drive their force as explained in the classics. Imagine roots branching out and down 3 feet or more into the earth from the "bubbling well" point on your foot with roots that are deep, strong, and flexible.

Is your Energy Circulating Freely and Smoothly?

This is a requirement and will be helped by you if you relax, be calm, relax your muscles thereby releasing tension in the body and mind. Maintain your structure and relax. Use the mindfulness to be aware of your body inside and out.

Are you Centered all the Time?

Being centered is a requirement and part of your foundational training and must continue in your practice. Remember Zhong Ding also called central equilibrium, is one of the keys in push hands and the mastery of Taiji.

Does everything move as one in unison?

If not then practice with the idea when one part moves everything moves and all moves as one unit. Then remember you must be able to move the chain a link at a time and stay connected. Is everything coordinated, inner and outer, above and below, mind and body? All should be in harmony and in unison.

Are you Song

One must be Song all the time. This means calm, relaxed and sunk having central equilibrium. When I touch you do I feel the ground? Do you have Peng jin? Have you become like a needle (how well do you neutralize)?

Have You Become the Ball

Have you become the ball? Do you have springy force? Remember the ball turns and does not allow anyone to penetrate its center. Key is relaxation, rooting and central equilibrium. Press against the ball and its relaxed springy force will throw you out.

Checklist of Advanced Practice Tips

- ✓ Insure that you are calm and your breath is even and deep all the time throughout the form and when you are doing push hands or applications. Insure you are inhaling during your yin phase and exhaling during your yang phase.
- ✓ Focus and pay attention at all times because this will help you be mindful, and calm during your forms and push hands practice.
- ✓ Maintain concentration even though there are many things going on around you. Some people can't practice if they are distracted but one should focus on what you are doing.
- ✓ Remember to be relaxed, listening and prepared to discharge at any given opportunity.
- ✓ Remember mind centered on lower dantian or at the bottom of the feet.
- ✓ Stay centered and maintain central equilibrium.
- ✓ Allow the internal Taiji to come to the forefront

Grandmaster Lui Bao Yu and Author

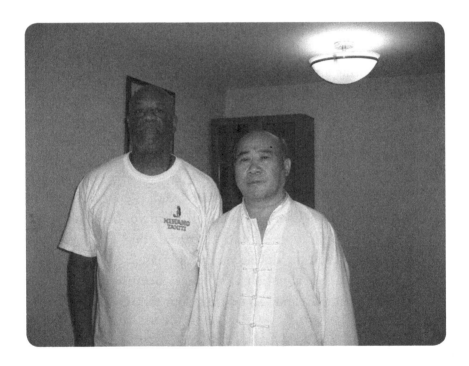

Master George Xu
Teaching Advanced Internal Sklls
Workshops at his Taiji Camps

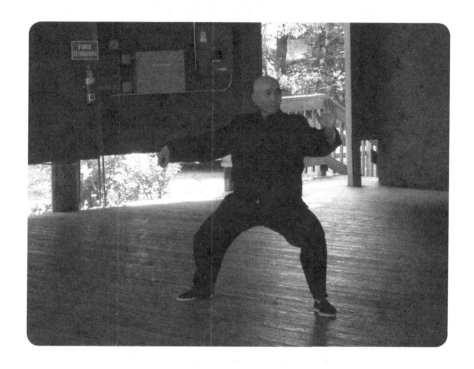

Basic Requirements of Advanced Skills and Techniques

Advanced skills and techniques are taught and learned after one has mastered the basic skills. The advanced skills require one to understand the skills of applications and how to practice at a higher level so that one can exhibit mastery of Taiji or internal martial arts. For example how does one incorporate the five elements within their practice and the higher skills of Taiji. For example, one should understand how the five elements are utilized such as fire, water, earth, metal, and air. How do you incorporate space dimension and moving from a place of the purely external to a place of purely internal. Understanding that the internal goes first then the external follows, until you reach the level of pure internal. Are you in total harmony with the internally and externally.

Cultivation of Consciousness

One must understand their own consciousness and how it has changed since one has developed higher Taiji skills and techniques. The consciousness changes just as our energy changes, grows, expands and refines itself. The consciousness of a beginner and a master practitioner is not the same hopefully. For those who are not clear the mind represents the consciousness and as one knows or has learned is that the mind (consciousness) is the commander and energy is the ruler. As one cultivates their consciousness they are at the same time cultivating their energy. As far as the body goes it is following the consciousness intent and the energy. The consciousness at this point is in full contact with all of its soldiers such as the legs, arms, fists and all other body parts. The consciousness is in harmony with the energy, the spirit and vitality of the practitioner. The spirit is operating and is focusing on taking one higher in the refinement of the art. This is a new experience for some and it is like the universe is expanding or opening to a new experience. One must begin to be aware of this refinement just as they are aware of the cultivation of their energy.

Advanced Skills and Techniques

Are you in harmony (six harmonies) with the internal and external? Beyond this there are many advanced skills that one can learn that focuses on an advanced understanding of the art of Taiji and the refinement of higher consciousness. Some you have to be careful within your practice especially with a partner and others that will help you to understand the philosophy of higher-level martial art. So what are a few of the higher advanced skills that one exhibits at the advanced and mastery level besides push hands:

- Dantian gong
- Fajin
- Dong jin
- Empty force or Ling Kong Jin
- Appearing, disappearing
- Advanced Spiral (tornado) training
- Third leg
- Third hand
- Gathering earth and heaven power
- Use of Third, Fourth and eight dimensional power
- Expanding and shrinking
- Space power
- Reducing enemies force to zero near and far
- Stopping opponents force from afar
- Pure internal
- Suck and swallow
- Expand and contract
- Transform change
- Superior force
- Superior power
- Healing others
- Dim Mak

Insight

Most of these skills are beyond basic skills and require learning with the assistance of a Master Teacher and the ability to practice with others to hone your skills. Some of these skills require you to learn how to function using these skills and techniques. Focus first on the basic and intermediate skills and techniques before you explore more advanced ones. There is no limit to learning but it requires dedication and an expansion of our consciousness along with a Master to tutor you properly. These skills are not just for fighting but are a part of moving toward the expression of the art of Taijiquan as a higher martial art.

Taiji Master *Chen Song-Tso and Author*

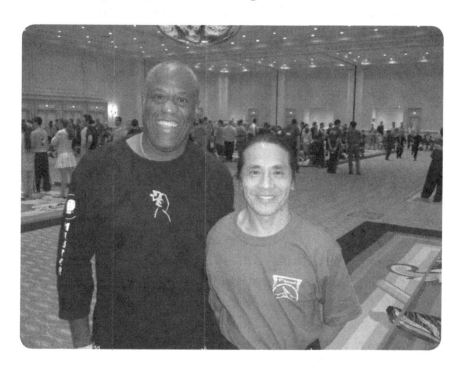

Insights from High Level Masters

On Rooting

Chen Zhaopi, the 18th generation Chen family master and master of Chen Xiao Wang, Chen Zhenglei, Chen Shitong, and Wang Xian, said the following: "If one cannot come to recognize how the weight moves distinctly back and forth between the two legs, then the upper and lower body cannot work together and connect. If the upper and lower body cannot connect, then you cannot absorb the opponent's force. If you cannot absorb the opponent's force, you cannot use his force."

Insight

This means if you cannot root and connect to the Earth's energy then you will not be able to absorb the opponent's force and not be able to deliver your own force.

Chen Pin-san, a great master of the 16th generation of the Chen family, once said, "Practice ten thousand reps, and you will come to understand Taijiquan." Grand master Chen Fa-ke practiced 30 reps a day throughout most of his life. Wu style Taijiquan founder Wu jian-quan asked his students to try to do ten thousands reps in three years. Master Chen Zhao-kui (son of Chen Fa-ke) said, "The practice of the form is the most important foundation work because the form is the end result of the accumulative fighting experience.

How to train your spirit and energy to drive the body

(Excerpt by Ren Gang by courtesy of www.doubledragonalliance.com)

Many people have already tried to explain what Taiji is, and what makes this art so special or different from other Chinese martial arts. Some translate it as "The Supreme Ultimate Fist" – giving students an idea that it is a great fighting art, based on strength, speed or martial skills.

But to Ren Gang, who is a long time student of Master Dong Bin of Shanghai China; its origins and explanation must be traced back to the concept of "Wu Ji" or "a state of emptiness", that is before Yin and Yang separate. Master Dong understood this principle and more importantly could utilize it, and one felt that he used no physical effort in deflecting an attacker, only Qi (energy) or "ling kong jin" (empty power).

Master Dong also knew many "shou fa" (martial applications) and just seemed like an encyclopedia of Taiji and Wushu. He believes very strongly that practitioners should follow the classic texts and principles carefully and try to find the meanings within their own bodies and feelings. People certainly shouldn't suspect or try to change the meanings within the texts as he has heard some teachers do. He said if you want to know if your practice is on track, you should check yourself. If you've spent a short amount of time practicing and have made lots of progress then you know you're right. But, if after practicing several years, you cannot push with or do well against an opponent who has practiced the same amount of time in other arts, then something must be wrong. You need to know where you're wrong and be able to address the problem. He said many people say that Taiji takes years to learn and so they say don't expect quick results. However he feels this is misleading. The honing and refining of Taiji skills has indeed no end, it is a lifelong study and not something that one can perfect in a few years, but one should be able to see definite progress inside three to five years.

What the practitioner should do is, at the point where the opponent is striking towards, one must "hua" or dissipate his potential force, where he is yang, you must be yin. But this apparent yielding or dissipating is not becoming "diu" or lost and lacking in substance, or "ruan" soft like tofu; it is accepting and welcoming his force like letting the wind blew through and out. Then your strike (yang) can fill the opponent's yin or weak place, now that his strength and force have been diffused. The adversary's energy is now completely spent, because you have emptied out his strong yang part by dissipating it. He becomes weak and unstable and empty. This concept of emptying out his force is called "yin jin luo kong" in Chinese. At this time, when he is completely empty and weak, you can issue power, "fajin".

One can only successfully issue power when the opponent is truly empty; otherwise if he is still strong and stable it becomes force against force.

When you issue, you must be able to release all your neng liang (內量(energy) to the opponent. Your body must be "tong tou" (通透) empty and almost transparent inside, with no tense places. To be "tong tou" we must first be "song" (relaxed) says Ren. But people often have a mistaken view of what "song" or relaxed means.

They know that being hard or tense is wrong but they then go to the other extreme and become "ruan" soft and collapsed in structure. This he says is an even bigger mistake. Like this, one can still not be truly relaxed and one loses one's own "neng li" the body's integrated and unified structural strength.

If one is just soft, one cannot use Taiji as a martial art, it just suffices as exercise. This is why many other disciplines scorn Taiji as a fighting system, because of this misunderstanding of "song" relaxed.

The body must be turned into a flowing, free-moving entity where one can move in an even, nimble and alive state. Some people like to imagine their bodies move like water, as this conjures up this feeling, but he says to move like air is an even better analogy. When one is genuinely relaxed, one cannot only move smoothly, quickly and naturally to deal with the opponent, but one can face life's challenges easily too.

Sometimes, new practitioners will feel that their body or hips etc. are not in the right position, and thus they will feel that their own bones are holding them back; at this juncture it's very hard to use one's shen Qi (energy). Once your body postures are correct you can start to move freely and you will start to discover your shen Qi. In Chinese, the waist eventually becomes an energetic center of the body, not a physical muscular or skeletal center.

At the outset, when one begins learning, students will treat the waist as a physical entity, which they will turn and move using bone and muscle, but this is a preliminary stage. The heart "Xin" first decides what to do and tells the waist, (this second energetic center or second heart and mind) and the waist then controls the energetic field or shen Qi and the shen Qi moves the rest of the body.

He said that this concept of the waist is not easy for beginners to grasp, but over years of practice one can obtain this feeling of it being a non-physical center. Without this sensation, he says he would not be able to smoothly and effortlessly remove an attacker's grab to his throat or body.

If he said, he treated his waist as a hard or physical place, then an attack on his throat in particular, would cause him to tense up and try to resist, thus allowing the attacker to gain an even stronger hold. When the waist moves, the legs and feet should follow the waist; this is what the principle of the waist being the commander means.

So what is "shen Qi"? When somebody practices Taiji form, they will slowly get a feeling that as they move, the air and energy around them is moving with them. (Taiji is often described as swimming in air.) Later one will feel that one is moving within an energy field, that one is connected to the surrounding environment, and that they can control and move this energy all around them. This energy is shen Qi. To explain more about the different types of energy connected to the body, Chinese says

"Gu rou de neng liang shi li liang, jing shen de neng liang shi shen Qi".

Basically translated, it just means that physical strength (liliang力量) is the expression or manifestation of energy (nengliang能量) from the physical body (gurou), and an invisible but yet tangible feeling of energy surrounding a person (shenQi神气) is the manifestation of the (jingshen精神) spirit's energy.

When you meet somebody who is usually quite strong and energetic, but who at that time is ill, you will feel that they have no vital force, no shenQi, so you do not feel intimidated or afraid of them, and are able to overcome them.

He says this kind of invisible energy force and spirit is what drives the body's movements, not your physical structure that carries out the movements.

In Taiji we should constantly try to practice, develop and enhance this shen Qi. In doing so, one will also change not just one's physical movements but one's character as well. The more relaxed one becomes, the greater their shenQi will be and the more generous, calm and open one will become.

He said this sense of calmness is a fundamental part of tuishou (push hands), fighting, or life in general. In push hands or sanshou (sparring) one must be calm and still inside. You must allow the opponent to fully take up his position or stance. Let him show you what he intends to do, this way you can clearly see where his faults and weaknesses are, thereby allowing you to take advantage of them and overcome him. If you act as most people do and immediately try to go against him or react out of anxiety or impatience the moment he opposes you, then you and he become locked in a battle, the outcome of which rests on the big overcoming the small, the strong overcoming the weak, or the fast defeating the slow. None of which are part of Taiji's internal principles.

In English we use one word to mean "emptiness", but in Chinese the idea of empty or nothing has many different meanings:

"KONG" – empty or free

"DIU" – empty, lost or without any firm structure or spirit

"MEI YOU" – without, nothing, don't have

So the problem for foreign students learning Wushu or the Chinese language itself is how to understand what real emptiness is, as in the state of "Wu Ji". We must realize that emptiness is not just nothing, but that it is emptiness and fullness combined. It is nothing and everything in complete harmony.

Before one moves, thinks, talks etc., one is first empty – wuji. An integrated whole which is in complete harmony with its surroundings. So, wu ji is in fact a quiet balanced state, where one thing exists peacefully and in harmony with another. In push hands or sparring etc., one must first look upon the opponent not as a separate entity that you must defeat – The Enemy – but as a part of you, a part of your energy circle.

Chinese philosophy looks upon a person as being as one with the earth and sky; they are in harmony not separate. If you can fully realize this and have a sensation of this state, than you can cultivate the feeling that the opponent is also one with you. But, it's not just his physical body that is one with you, his spirit and "shen Qi" vital energy around him, is part of your energy sphere too. So in Taiji, we want to first become aware of and later be able to harness this shen Qi.

Often people play the form and have a feeling of energy moving the body's structure, but as soon as they push hands with someone, they go back to using physical strength or their structure, and are more concerned about winning and thus lose control of their shen Qi.

In "Nei Jia Quan" internal arts, like Taiji, we want to forget about the body's structure and strength and utilize the shen Qi to move our own body and deal with the opponent.

In Chinese they say the "xin" heart or unconscious thought controls your waist, the waist controls and moves the shen qi and your shen qi moves the physical body. If you want to do something, you feel what it is you want to do, and then your body responds. You must train yourself to use your heart (Xin) and waist to control your shen qi and thus change your old habits of the physical body or your rational thought moving the energy.

He said that when one moves, whatever one wants to do or decides to do, the body will just follow precisely what you intend. In push hands, when you see the opportunity to dissipate or strike the opponent, your body immediately obeys this "thought" or feeling with action. He said if you have to wrestle and struggle to try and overcome the opponent to move him, then this is wrong.

At first, Ren mentioned, your body won't listen to your intention or your waist, but over time, as you concentrate on this aspect, you will start to cultivate a sensation. Finally I asked him about his hopes for the future of Taiji.

He said if he ever reaches a stage where he understands the secrets of Taiji and can use them, then he would certainly want to share this knowledge with everyone, so that all lovers of Taiji can share in the splendor of this wonderful art. Finally, he reiterated, that you must be open and generous in spirit. Your shen Qi (an energy field that surrounds you and is interconnected with your spirit) and your "Qi liang" (generosity of spirit) is connected, so if you're a mean person your shen Qi will also be small, and you'll be able to utilize very little of this force.

Insight

The idea of learning from masters and teachers is important because they have went through the path you are trying to follow and can help guide you on your way. Fortunately we can glean vital insight from others who are practicing the art of Taijiquan. The excerpts are to give you insight from different perspectives, which is important when one is trying to gain insight and grow in their practice. Also it is important when trying to correct and refine your practice especially without the benefit of a Master Teacher. The advice given is to be read and digested so that you can measure where you are and what you need to grow. The classics can guide you but you must put in the practice.

Practicing Hunyuan Qigong with
Grandmaster Feng Zhiqiang in China

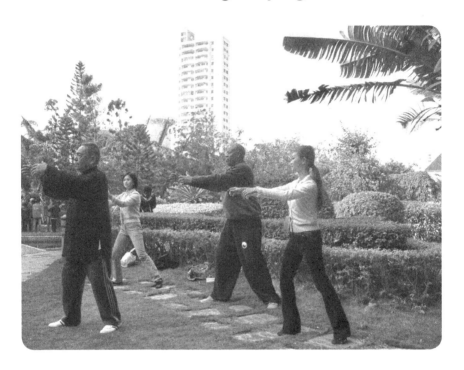

A Note from Grandmaster Feng ZhiQiang's important teachings:

Standing gong practice

Feng emphasizes the standing gong practice greatly. He points out that this simple training method holds the key to Taiji power and energy. He says students should do a lot of standing gong, and they should do it in a calm and relaxed manner. According to Feng, standing gong is the soul of Taiji.

Slow form practice

Feng considers slow form practice as better practice. He says slow practice nurtures your Qi, improves your health and increases your power in self-defense. According to Feng, too much fajin and fast form training actually can have a debilitating effect on your health and energy. You should practice your Taiji form as slow as possible, but without struggle.

Looseness in Chen Taiji

Looseness, or song in Chinese, is an important aspect of Chen Style. Feng says some people think "song" is unimportant in Chen Style. This is a wrong concept. It is not easy to be "song" while practicing the form, but students should try very hard to relax. Without the element of "song", it will be impossible to enter the threshold of Taiji.

About turning – silk-reeling

Silk reeling, or turning, is crucial to good Chen Taiji practice. All parts of the body should have silk-reeling property. This is the key to what the classic called "to use 4 oz. to move a thousand lbs.". Silk-reeling exercises are the high-level of gong training in Chen style. The ability of rotating any parts of one's body like a ball is the key to avoiding double heaviness, or fighting force with force.

Nurturing

Feng puts the concept of nurturing at the top of his list. Once while being interviewed by a Chinese magazine, he said. "After decades of Taiji practice, I finally realize one word – nurturing." He also said, "In a ten years practice, you should nurture your Qi and body for ten years." Nurturing is good for both health and martial art.

Insight

There are many roads to mastering the art of Taiji. Some are straight paths that take less time. Others are crooked roads that take forever. Master Feng once said, "Famous teachers might not be illuminating teachers." An illuminating teaches a straight path; and a straight path is the path with the least detours. In this sense, I can say Feng is a real grandmaster and an illuminating teacher.

The theory workshop concentrates on the following 8 unique characteristic features of Chen-style Taijiquan:

- Conscious movements under command of the brain (Yi).
- The springy movements by lengthening the different parts of the body.
- The forward and backward diametrically opposed spiraling movements.
- The substantial and insubstantial movements under the requirements of an upright straight torso and the complete co-ordination of all body parts.
- The chain actions led by the waist and the full synchronization of internal/external.

- Uninterrupted, smooth and magnificent Yangtze River water-like movements.
- The processing of softness to hardness and hardness to softness and the correct combination.
- From slower to quicker, and to slower, the different speeds of practicing in the different learning stages. The different speed of movements in Chen-style Taijiquan.

The Five Essentials for Victory
(**Reference: Sun Tzu Chapter 3**: Attach by Stratagem Translated by Lionel Giles)

Thus we may know that there are five essentials for victory:

(1)   He will win who knows when to fight and when not to fight.
(2)   He will win who knows how to handle both superior and inferior forces.
(3)   He will win whose army is animated by the same spirit throughout all its ranks.
(4)   He will win who, prepared himself, waits to take the enemy unprepared.
(5)   He will win who has military capacity and is not interfered with by the sovereign.

Hence the saying: If you know the enemy and know yourself, you need not fear the result of a hundred battles. If you know yourself but not the enemy, for every victory gained you will also suffer a defeat. If you know neither the enemy nor yourself, you will succumb in every battle.

Yang's Ten Important Points

(by Yang Cheng-fu (1883 - 1936)

1.) 虛靈頂勁Head upright to let the shen (spirit of vitality) rise to the top of the head. Don't use li [external strength], or the neck will be stiff and the ch'i (vital life energy) and blood cannot flow through. It is necessary to have a natural and lively feeling. If the spirit cannot reach the head top, it cannot raise.

2.) 含胸拔背Sink the chest and pluck up the back. The chest is depressed naturally inward so that the ch'i can sink to the dantian (field of elixir). Don't expand the chest: the ch'i gets stuck there and the body becomes top-heavy. The heel will be too light and can be uprooted. Pluck up the back and the ch'i sticks to the back; depress the chest and you can pluck up the back. Then you can discharge force through the spine. You will be a peerless boxer.

3.) 鬆腰Sung [Relax] the waist. The waist is the commander of the whole body. If you can sung the waist, then the two legs will have power and the lower part will be firm and stable. Substantial and insubstantial change, and this is based on the turning of the waist. It is said "the source of the postures lies in the waist. If you cannot get power, seek the defect in the legs and waist."

4.) 虛實分明Differentiate between insubstantial and substantial. This is the first principle in Taijiquan. If the weight of the whole body is resting on the right leg, then the right leg is substantial and the left leg is insubstantial, and vice versa. When you can separate substantial and insubstantial, you can turn lightly without using strength. If you cannot separate, the step is heavy and slow. The stance is not firm and can be easily thrown of balance.

5.) 沈肩墜肘Sink the shoulders and drop the elbows. The shoulders will be completely relaxed and open. If you cannot relax and sink, the two shoulders will be raised up and tense. The ch'i will follow them up and the whole body cannot get power. "Sink the elbows" means the elbows go down and relax. If the elbows raise, the shoulders are not able to sink and you cannot discharge people far. The discharge will then be close to the broken force of the external schools.

6.) 用意不用力Use the mind instead of force. The Taijiquan Classics say, "all of this means use I [mind-intent] and not li." In practicing Taijiquan the whole body relaxes. Don't let one ounce of force remain in the blood vessels, bones, and ligaments to tie yourself up. Then you can be agile and able to change. You will be able to turn freely and easily. Doubting this, how can you increase your power?

The body has meridians like the ground has ditches and trenches. If not obstructed the water can flow. If the meridian is not closed, the ch'i goes through. If the whole body has hard force and it fills up the meridians, the ch'i and the blood stop and the turning is not smooth and agile. Just pull one hair and the whole body is off-balance. If you use I, and not li, then the I goes to a place in the body and the Qi follows it. The ch'i and the blood circulate. If you do this every day and never stop, after a long time you will have nei Jin [real internal strength]. The Taijiquan Classics say, "when you are extremely soft, you become extremely hard and strong." Someone who has extremely good Taijiquan kungfu has arms like iron wrapped with cotton and the weight is very heavy. As for the external schools, when they use li, they reveal li. When they don't use li, they are too light and floating. Their chin is external and locked together. The li of the external schools is easily led and moved, and not too be esteemed.

7.) 上下相隨Coordinate the upper and lower parts of the body. The Taijiquan Classics say, "the motion should be rooted in the feet, released through the legs, controlled by the waist and manifested through the fingers." Everything acts simultaneously. When the hand, waist and foot move together, the eyes follow. If one part doesn't follow, the whole body is disordered.

8.) 內外相合Harmonize the internal and external. In the practice of Taijiquan the main thing is the spirit. Therefore it is said "the spirit is the commander and the body is subordinate." If you can raise the spirit, then the movements will naturally be agile. The postures are not beyond insubstantial and substantial, opening and closing. That which is called open means not only the hands and feet are open, but also the mind is also open. That which is called closed means not only the hands and feet are closed, but the mind is also closed. When you can make the inside and outside become one, then it becomes complete.

9.) 連绵不斷Move with continuity. As to the external schools, their chin is the Latter Heaven brute chin. Therefore it is finite. There are connections and breaks. During the breaks the old force is exhausted and the new force has not yet been born. At these moments it is very easy for others to take advantage. Taijiquan uses I and not li. From beginning to end it is continuous and not broken. It is circular and again resumes. It revolves and has no limits. The original Classics say it is "like a great river rolling on unceasingly." and that the circulation of the Jin is "drawing silk from a cocoon " They all talk about being connected together.

10.) 動中求靜Move with tranquility [Seek stillness in movement]. The external schools assume jumping about is good and they use all their energy. That is why after practice everyone pants. Taijiquan uses stillness to control movement. Although one moves, there is also stillness. Therefore in practicing the form, slower is better. If it is slow, the inhalation and exhalation are long and deep and the Qi sinks to the dantian (丹田). Naturally there is no injurious practice such as engorgement of the blood vessels. The learner should be careful to comprehend it. Then you will get the real meaning.

Chen GrandMaster Zhu Xiang Qian

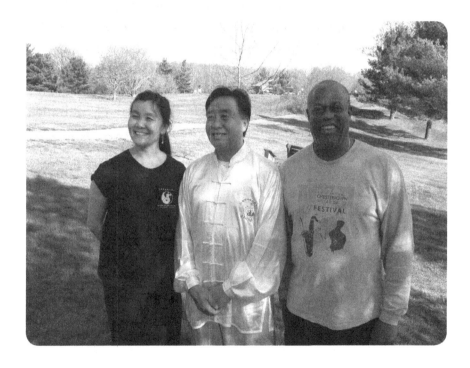

Always Becoming the Master

Always becoming the master implies that you have as a goal to master the art of Taijiquan, and you want to go beyond the weekend warrior practitioner and you are dedicated to learning and mastering the art on some high level above novice. This also implies that you are dedicated to this art and practice and will do what is required to reach a high level and eventually teach and/or share your knowledge and experiences with others on the same path as you. This contract with yourself pushes you to study, research, practice, preserve, go beyond basics and focus on improving yourself and your practice as much as possible. This also implies that you love the art and are learning for the sake of the art. This also requires much study and practice and learning also from a qualified teacher or master if at all possible. This also includes the practice of the forms, weapons, push hands and higher-level practices of cultivation including the energetic and spiritual understanding of the internal art.

Right Teacher Right Student

It is important to understand that the art of Taiji requires the assistant of a Teacher as the best way to master the art of Taiji. If you have a Taiji master as your teacher you are in the best place, right time to take advantage of this gift and learn as much as possible. Many people do not have the opportunity such as a teacher. This also must require you to be the right student. Being the right student requires a few of the following attributes:

- Listening
- Open to learning
- Emptying the full glass
- Practicing and perseverance
- Trust
- Doing research
- Study

- Not challenging the Teacher
- Asking questions at the appropriate time

Becoming a Teacher, Master and or Grandmaster

What is a Teacher?

A teacher is a dedicated practitioner who has turned to impart knowledge and experience to those who want to learn the art of Taiji and become internal martial artists of the art.

A Teacher should have the following qualities:

- Skill level – must have a high skill level of the art.
- Knowledge – must have considerable knowledge of the art.
- Willingness to teach others.
- WuDe (武德) respect for the students and the proper character

Can one become a Master?

Yes one can become a master. Some Masters say no, some say yes. I say yes you can, it is possible if you are dedicated, has help from a knowledgeable Master who is willing to share his knowledge and wisdom, also help from within and assistance from the Higher Source. It also will require a level of dedication on your part and help from your Taiji brothers and sisters. It also requires one refine their consciousness, to open to the universal.

What is a Master?

A master is a dedicated practitioner of the art of internal martial arts such as Taijiquan. One who has extensive knowledge and can demonstrate that in-depth knowledge of the art he or she practices. A master is one who has extensive experience and who understands the many levels within the art and who has mastered the art in some way or fashion to be deemed a master. A master of internal martial arts can demonstrate form and function of the art and who is dedicated to its practice, the sharing of that knowledge and the promotion of the art via writings, teaching or spreading the art form itself via competitions or seminars or workshops.

A Master should have the following qualities:

- Skill level – must have an extremely high skill level of the art.
- Knowledge – must have deep knowledge of the art.
- Contribution – must contribute something to sharing his knowledge of the art.
- Dedication – must dedicate much of his time and effort to the same art.

What is a Grandmaster?

A grandmaster is one who has mastered the art of internal martial arts and helped develop masters. One who can demonstrate the art, one who has taught the art and spread the art by sharing their knowledge of the art with their students, other teachers or masters, the general public at large and promotes the entire system such as Taijiquan. Listed below are some of the qualities of a Grandmaster.

Qualities of a Grandmaster

A Grandmaster should have the following qualities:

- Skill level – must have an extremely high skill level of the art.
- Knowledge – must have deep knowledge of the art.
- Seniority – must be high in the lineage, therefore quite old.
- Contribution – must contribute something to improve the art.

- Dedication – must dedicate much of his time and effort to the same art.

These are the qualifications of a grandmaster.

Note: A Grandmaster is someone very special; he or she is one of the supreme teachers of the style or branch.

Insight

Not all students are good students with good character. I have taught some who did not represent WuDe and I have heard many stories of bad students. Not all teachers are created alike. Some teachers can teach, some are not that skilled and like students, teachers should understand WuDe (武德) also. Teachers should have good character but all are not the same so one should look to a proper teacher with good character and a willingness to teach.

One should not give up on trying to master the art even if you cannot find a master teacher to assist you. Persevere and it will happen. Learn, practice, study, and research. This will help you grow toward your goal. Remember a glass full cannot accept any more water.

Being a master or grandmaster is a great responsibility because one is representing the art that has been passed down from generations to generations and those who are masters and grandmasters of the high art love the art and want to see it grow and prosper in a positive direction globally. So respectfully it requires us to pay homage to those past Masters and the current ones representing the art for arts' sake. Respect those who have come to share their knowledge and wisdom. Remember WuDe (武德), which is important for all students and teachers to respect the traditions, the culture, the treasure and the ancestors. Chinese martial artists have a saying: "A student will spend three years looking for a good teacher, and a teacher will test a student for three years."

Song of Longevity

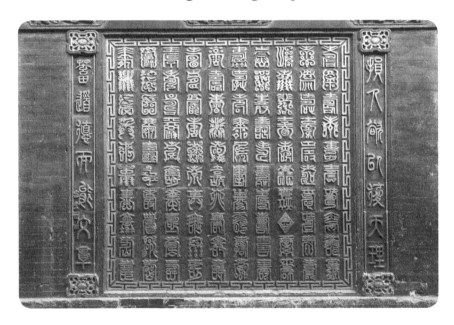

Mysterious to the Miraculous (Shen Ming)

The Spiritual Aspects

Taijiquan requires self-cultivation, which at the higher levels means attainment. We have mentioned the refinement of consciousness and the necessary self-cultivation of the mind and energy but this includes the heart also. The spiritual aspects of the art of Taiji cannot be negated or neglected as one rises to the level of master. It is told that in order to rise up to a level of mastery one must be able to include the heart and mind. What does love have to do with it? It is also important to understand that love of the art is required in order to advance to a level of mastery. Also the highest level of the art is a rise to the level of going beyond self and is considered to be a spiritual practice because one is at the level of being not only inside of the door of Taiji which means you are doing an internal practice and you have settled to the point of practicing for the sake of the art. But one has raised his or her consciousness and is thinking about the Dao, the way, the universe and what else is there. You should be at a point of thinking about the inner peace one is feeling or experiencing. This is a higher level of thought that is not limited by their environment or surroundings and they are continuing their inner cultivation (neizai xiujyang 内在修养.) Understanding the time, space continuum and the Dao is part of advanced skills that are part of the higher art.

One other aspect one should consider is the healing aspects of the art and the healing of others within their spear of influence. This higher level thought process inspired by the heart and Shen moves one beyond the daily momentary grind of basic practice or fighting to the universal aspects of helping, healing, sharing, teaching, loving the art and realizing they are part of the One whole spiritual universe. While at the same time thinking about longevity of life and the universal.

As one says at this level, I reach the top of the mountain and complete my journey, I turn and see a mountain higher and I am ready to complete the next journey. I also turn and look back to see whom I can help or assist that is making the same journey. The earth is at my feet, the heavens are within reach as my head is above, and I am connected to the one and the all!

What is happening inside that no one can see is important such are you are upset, angry, stressed, depressed or are you smiling? There is something called the inner smile and as a master one should be smiling inside and there should be cultivation within of peace and happiness that brings us to smiling because we know and are happy. So work on your inner smile and teach your students to smile within. Remember the visible becomes the invisible so even if you cannot see, it does not mean it cannot and did not happen. Miracles do happen so look for the miracles in your life from this ultimate practice of this High art. Also there are advanced techniques not readily available for the novice and so many of the hidden techniques require advanced understanding and knowledge garnered from ones' practice or from their Teacher. Some are discussed and practiced when one is ready to move beyond the basics and intermediate, ready to understand the more ultimate advanced skills that masters keep hidden for various reasons. Remember when one is ready the Teacher will appear or go search for them.

Insight

I will explain only that at the higher levels the practice of Taijiquan is an art and so the consciousness of the practitioner has changed. The understanding of mind-intent, will, energy, perception, view of the opponent and the world has changed. Your perception of martial arts has changed from the in-look to the outlook and how one affects the macrocosm. The understanding of how you affect others has changed and you now have progressed passed the attack and defend physiological and psychological approaches you once used. One now focuses on the human character and its transformation. The thought process now focuses on life, longevity and the Dao.

At this level one focuses on Taiji as an art and one realizes you are not alone and are at one within your heart and one with the universal. It is the realization of the Ultimate. Contemplate what is next for you as you become the master! Practice your inner smile while you are practicing the art. A master painter paints because that is what is in their heart and mind the same place where love resides. Healing is a part of mastery and one should utilize their cultivated skills to help heal themselves, teach others, and help heal others in order to promote the art and treasure of Taiji. As you reach higher levels of attainment within your practice you should focus on the spiritual, internal and the Dao.

Grandmaster Zhu Xiang Qian, Master C.P. Ong Chen Workshop

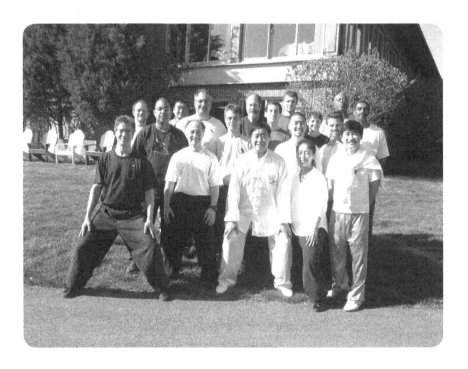

More Insight on My Journey

I have traveled the world, learned many things, Taiji forms, skills, insights, secrets and have much more to learn. The best part is the knowledge and experiences I have received from my Teachers, Masters, Taiji brothers and sisters from around the world. Some learning, some experienced, some experts on the path, some having reached the pinnacle of success and all have said they are in the way (Dao) and I am doing the same.

I have learned that the path is the journey, the experiences are the flowers, and the interactions, the glances left and right that we see as we pass on the road to success. I ignore the small rocks (obstacles) on the side of the road. The mountain is before me and I have climbed many and met many a Master who has kept the promise of being an example for many to follow and happy I passed their way. It is our vision that leads us to the door of success, our tenacity to walk through it unafraid as to what is on the other side and our open hearts to empty the glass and learn more than we envision but like fresh roses we keep growing. It is impossible to reach the top of the mountain if you are afraid to climb or refuse to learn from the one who has went before you up to the top of the mountain. It takes practice, perseverance, and knowing that you can succeed if you are willing to stick with it but it is also good to be you and practice the art at any level you choose to be. Water seeks its own level so you can go as deep as you care to or stay at the shallow end of the pool. We are all still swimming in the ocean of this treasure and are the better for it. This path of the ultimate includes creating practitioners cultivating higher consciousness so they can demonstrate the higher levels of internal arts.

I continue to play even when I was a child and now as an adult and will continue as an ancient because the child in your lives on and continues to grow in the DAO. Remember the sun shines everyday as the earth moves forward turning to meet you in the way (DAO) so as we practice the art of Taiji on the earth the heavens tap us on the head to let us know we are in the grand ultimate (Taijiquan). Sharing our experiences, knowledge and wisdom is part of our destiny to help the others. As a Chinese Master once said me, "to be friends from unlikely places can unite the world when we see all as brothers and sisters as one huge global family."

If you have an opportunity travel to the centers of Wushu and Internal martial arts in China, Hong Kong, and Taiwan for self-immersion it is worth it. If you want to really understand why millions who love the art and practice it everyday go for a visit.

I have grown and now realize that I must also help those who want to also grow. I treasure each pearl I gain as I practice the art of Taijiquan. I see growth each day so I know I am on the right track and must continue on my journey. As far as the remarkable everyday is a day to experience the remarkable so be open to learning the ultimate and remember when you reach the top of the mountain turn and see the new mountain in front of you and turn to help someone trying to make the climb. One is always learning even as they are teaching, so continue to grow. Keep on cultivating to the higher consciousness. Let's practice this treasure we call Taijiquan as an art. We are always becoming the master.

Bodhidharma

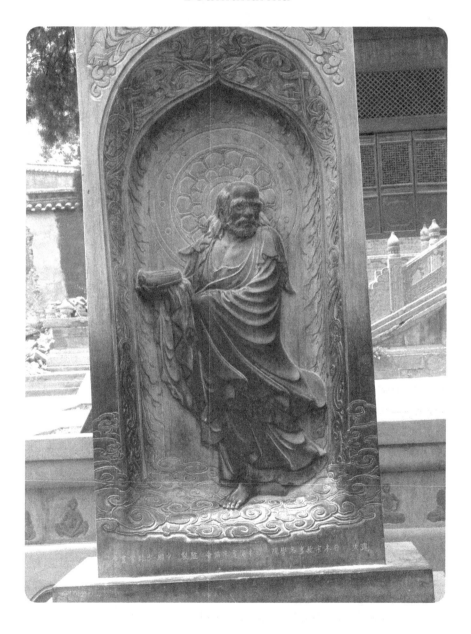

My Song of Taiji Gong
By George Samuels

I turned to the left as I saw the right
I lifted up after sinking down
Spiraled to my left
Then to my right
Gave a little so I could receive as
I warded off and pulled the opponent down
Only for them to reverse as I reversed first

I sunk looking for the energy
As the sky above me touched my head
Letting me know I was centered and connected
I realized the spiral on the end of my hand was endless
As I turned to meet the sky and lifted up the cloud
It was clear that I extend and then shrink
Until they gave in
And I exposed the center of him as I hid

Looking for new light and the way in
The energy surged as I sunk
The waves swayed back and forth
To the left and right
As I stay centered
And the paddles turn left and right
To support the change
From yin to yang

I am comfortable as I relax
Sink and circulate like a tree
As he grabs my branch and I allow
The branches of my bamboo to sway and spring back
Sending the opponent flying high

As the wind blows the boat to a distant shore
Comfortable with the calm of the sea
And the sun rising to meet the day
I sigh knowing I am Song, at peace in my heart, and focused
On the universe and me
Ready, all in unison to meet the new day
As I practice anew my ultimate Taiji Gong
In a new way!

Tortoise of longevity

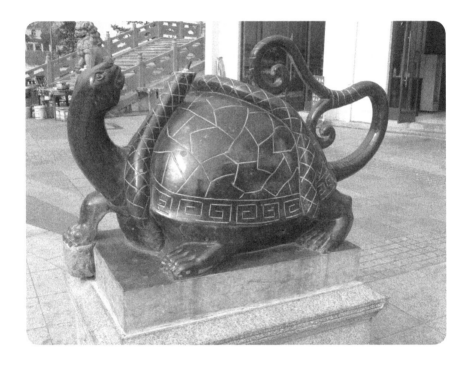

The Neijia Inner Cultivation or Inward Training

Author unknown (4th century) Translated by Harold Roth

One

The vital essence of all things:
It is this that brings them to life.
It generates the five grains below
And becomes the constellated stars above.
When flowing amid the heavens and the earth
We call it ghostly and numinous.
When stored within the chests of human beings,
We call them sages.

Two

Therefore this vital energy is:
Bright! - as if ascending from the heavens;
Dark! - as if entering an abyss;
Vast! - as if dwelling in an ocean;
Lofty! - as if dwelling on a mountain peak.
Therefore this vital energy
Cannot be halted by force,
Yet can be secured by inner power [Te].
Cannot be summoned by speech,
Yet can be welcomed by awareness.
Reverently hold onto it and do not lose it:
This is called "developing inner power."
When inner power develops and wisdom emerges,
The myriad things will, to the last one, be grasped.

Three

All the forms of the mind
Are naturally infused and filled with it [the vital essence],
Are naturally generated and developed [because of] it.
It is lost
Inevitably because of sorrow, happiness, joy, anger, desire, and profit
seeking.
If you are able to cast off sorrow, happiness, joy, anger, desire and
profit-seeking,
Your mind will just revert to equanimity.
The true condition of the mind
Is that it finds calmness beneficial and, by it, attains repose.
Do not disturb it, do not disrupt it
And harmony will naturally develop.

Four

Clear! as though right by your side.
Vague! as though it will not be attained.
Indescribable! as though beyond the limitless.
The test of this is not far off:
Daily we make use of its inner power.
The Way is what infuses the body,
Yet people are unable to fix it in place.
It goes forth but does not return,
It comes back but does not stay.
Silent! none can hear its sound.
Suddenly stopping! it abides within the mind.
Obscure! we do not see its form.
Surging forth! it arises with us.
We do not see its form,
We do not hear its sound,
Yet we can perceive an order to its accomplishments.
We call it "the Way."

Five

The Way has no fixed position;
It abides within the excellent mind.
When the mind is tranquil and the vital breath is regular,
The Way can thereby be halted.
That Way is not distant from us;
When people attain it they are sustained
That Way is not separated from us;
When people accord with it they are harmonious.
Therefore: Concentrated! as though you could be roped together with it.
Indiscernible! as though beyond all locations.
The true state of that Way:
How could it be conceived of and pronounced upon?
Cultivate your mind, make your thoughts tranquil,
And the Way can thereby be attained.

Six

As for the Way:
It is what the mouth cannot speak of,
The eyes cannot see,
And the ears cannot hear.
It is that with which we cultivate the mind and align the body.
When people lose it they die;
When people gain it they flourish.
When endeavors lose it they fail;
When they gain it they succeed.
The Way never has a root or trunk,
It never has leaves or flowers.
The myriad things are generated by it;
The myriad things are completed by it.
We designate it "the Way."

Seven

For the heavens, the ruling principle is to be aligned.
For the earth, the ruling principle is to be level.
For human beings the ruling principle is to be tranquil.
Spring, autumn, winter and summer are the seasons of the heavens.
Mountains, hills, rivers, and valleys are the resources of the earth.
Pleasure and anger, accepting and rejecting are the devices of human beings.
Therefore, the sage:
Alters with the seasons but doesn't transform,
Shifts with things but doesn't change places with them.

Eight

If you can be aligned and be tranquil,
Only then can you be stable.
With a stable mind at your core,
With the eyes and ears acute and clear,
And with the four limbs firm and fixed,
You can thereby make a lodging place for the vital essence.
The vital essence: it is the essence of the vital energy.
When the vital energy is guided, it [the vital essence] is generated,
But when it is generated, there is thought,
When there is thought, there is knowledge,
But when there is knowledge, then you must stop.
Whenever the forms of the mind have excessive knowledge,
You loose your vitality.

Nine

Those who can transform even a single thing, call them "numinous";
Those who can alter even a single situation, call them "wise."
But to transform without expending vital energy; to alter without expending wisdom:

Only exemplary persons who hold fast to the One are able to do this.
Hold fast to the One; do not loose it,
And you will be able to master the myriad things.
Exemplary persons act upon things,
And are not acted upon by them,
Because they grasp the guiding principle of the One.

Ten

With a well-ordered mind within you,
Well-ordered words issue forth from your mouth,
And well-ordered tasks are imposed on others.
Then all under heaven will be well ordered.
"When one word is grasped,
All under the heavens will submit.
When one word is fixed,
All under heavens will listen."
It is this [word "Way"] to which the saying refers.

Eleven

When your body is not aligned,
The inner power will not come.
When you are not tranquil within,
Your mind will not be ordered.
Align your body, assist the inner power,
Then it will gradually come on its own.

Twelve

The numinous [mind]: no one knows its limit;
It intuitively knows the myriad things.
Hold it within you, do not let it waver.
To not disrupt your senses with external things,

To not disrupt your mind with your senses:
This is called "grasping it within you."

Thirteen

There is a numinous [mind] naturally residing within;
One moment it goes, the next it comes,
And no one is able to conceive of it.
If you loose it you are inevitably disordered;
If you attain it you are inevitably well ordered.
Diligently clean out its lodging place
And its vital essence will naturally arrive.
Still your attempts to imagine and conceive of it.
Relax your efforts to reflect on and control it.
Be reverent and diligent
And its vital essence will naturally stabilize.
Grasp it and don't let go
Then the eyes and ears won't overflow
And the mind will have nothing else to seek.
When a properly aligned mind resides within you,
The myriad things will be seen in their proper perspective.

Fourteen

The Way fills the entire world.
It is everywhere that people are,
But people are unable to understand this.
When you are released by this one word:
You reach up to the heavens above;
You stretch down to the earth below;
You pervade the nine inhabited regions.
What does it mean to be released by it?
The answer resides in the calmness of the mind.
When your mind is well ordered, your senses are well ordered.

When your mind is calm, your senses are calmed.
What makes them well ordered is the mind;
What makes them calm is the mind.
By means of the mind you store the mind:
Within the mind there is yet another mind.
That mind within the mind: it is an awareness that precedes words.
Only after there is awareness does it take shape;
Only after it takes shape it there a word.
Only after there is a word is it implemented;
Only after it is implemented is there order.
Without order, you will always be chaotic.
If chaotic, you die.

Fifteen

For those who preserve and naturally generate vital essence
On the outside a calmness will flourish.
Stored inside, we take it to be the wellspring.
Flood-like, it harmonizes and equalizes
And we take it to be the fount of the vital energy.
When the fount is not dried up,
The four limbs are firm.
When the spring is not drained,
Vital energy freely circulates through the nine apertures.
You can then exhaust the heavens and the earth
And spread over the four seas.
When you have no delusions within you,
Externally there will be no disasters.
Those who keep their minds unimpaired within,
Externally keep their bodies unimpaired,
Who do not encounter heavenly disasters
Or meet with harm at the hands of others,
Call them Sages.

Sixteen

If people can be aligned and tranquil,
Their skin will be ample and smooth,
Their eyes and ears will be acute and clear,
Their muscles will be supple and their bones will be strong,
They will then be able to hold up the Great Circle [of the heavens]
And tread firmly over the Great Square [of the earth].
They will mirror things with great purity.
And they will perceive things with great clarity.
Reverently be aware [of the Way] and do not waver,
And you will daily renew your inner power,
Thoroughly understand all under the heavens,
And exhaust everything within the Four Directions.
To reverently bring forth the effulgence [of the Way]:
This is called "inward attainment."
If you do this but fail to return to it,
This will cause a wavering in your vitality.

Seventeen

For all [to practice] this Way:
You must coil, you must contract,
You must uncoil, you must expand,
You must be firm, you must be regular [in this practice].
Hold fast to this excellent [practice]; do not let go of it.
Chase away the excessive; abandon the trivial.
And when you reach its ultimate limit
You will return to the Way and the inner power.

Eighteen

When there is a mind that is unimpaired within you,
It cannot be hidden.

It will be known in your countenance,
And seen in your skin color.
If with this good flow of vital energy you encounter others,
They will be kinder to you than your own brethren.
But if with a bad flow of vital energy you encounter others,
They will harm you with their weapons.
[This is because] the wordless pronouncement
Is more rapid than the drumming of thunder.
The perceptible form of the mind's vital energy
Is brighter than the sun and moon,
And more apparent than the concern of parents.
Rewards are not sufficient to encourage the good;
Punishments are not sufficient to discourage the bad.
Yet once this flow of vital energy is achieved,
All under heaven will submit.
And once the mind is made stable,
All under heaven will listen.

Nineteen

By concentrating your vital breath as if numinous,
The myriad things will all be contained within you.
Can you concentrate? Can you unite with them?
Can you not resort to divining by tortoise or milfoil
Yet know bad and good fortune?
Can you stop? Can you cease?
Can you not seek it in others,
Yet attain it within yourself?
You think and think about it
And think still further about it.
You think, yet still cannot penetrate it.
While the ghostly and numinous will penetrate it,
It is not due to the power of the ghostly and numinous,
But to the utmost refinement of your essential vital breathe.

When the four limbs are aligned
And the blood and vital breath are tranquil,
Unify your awareness, concentrate your mind,
Then your eyes and ears will not be over-stimulated.
And even the far-off will seem close at hand.

Twenty

Deep thinking generates knowledge.
Idleness and carelessness generate worry.
Cruelty and arrogance generate resentment.
Worry and grief generate illness.
When illness reaches a distressing degree, you die.
When you think about something and don't let go of it,
Internally you will be distressed, externally you will be weak.
Do not plan things out in advance
Or else your vitality will cede its dwelling.
In eating, it is best not to fill up;
In thinking, it is best not to overdo.
Limit these to the appropriate degree
And you will naturally reach it [vitality].

Twenty-one

As for the life of all human beings:
The heavens brings forth their vital essence,
The earth brings forth their bodies.
These two combine to make a person.
When they are in harmony there is vitality;
When they are not in harmony there is no vitality.
If we examine the Way of harmonizing them,
Its essentials are not visible,
Its signs are not numerous.
Just let a balanced and aligned [breathing] fill your chest

And it will swirl and blend with your mind,
This confers longevity.
When joy and anger are not limited,
You should make a plan [to limit them].
Restrict the five sense-desires;
Cast away these dual misfortunes.
Be not joyous, be not angry,
Just let a balanced and aligned [breathing] fill your chest.

Twenty-two

As for the vitality of all human beings:
It inevitably occurs because of balanced and aligned [breathing].
The reason for its loss
Is inevitably pleasure and anger, worry and anxiety.
Therefore, to bring your anger to a halt, there is nothing better than poetry;
To cast off worry there is nothing better than music;
To limit music there is nothing better than rites;
To hold onto the rites there is nothing better than reverence;
To hold onto reverence there is nothing better than tranquility.
When you are inwardly tranquil and outwardly reverent
You are able to return to your innate nature
And this nature will become greatly stable.

Twenty-three

For all the Way of eating is that:
Overfilling yourself with food will impair your vital energy
And cause your body to deteriorate.
Over-restricting your consumption causes the bones to wither
And the blood to congeal.
The mean between overfilling and over-restricting:
This is called "harmonious completion."

It is where the vital essence lodges
And knowledge is generated.
When hunger and fullness lose their proper balance,
You make a plan to correct this.
When full, move quickly;
When hungry, neglect your thoughts;
When old, forget worry.
If when full you don't move quickly,
Vital energy will not circulate to your limbs.
If when hungry you don't neglect your thoughts of food,
When you finally eat you will not stop.
If when old you don't forget your worries,
The fount of your vital energy will rapidly drain out.

Twenty-four

When you enlarge your mind and let go of it,
When you relax your vital breath and expand it,
When your body is calm and unmoving:
And you maintain the One and discard the myriad disturbances,
You will see profit and not be enticed by it,
You will see harm and not be frightened by it.
Relaxed and unwound, yet acutely sensitive,
In solitude you delight in your own person.
This is called "revolving the vital breath":
Your thoughts and deeds seem heavenly.

Twenty-five

The vitality of all people
Inevitably comes from their peace of mind.
When anxious, you loose this guiding thread;
When angry, you lose this basic point.
When you are anxious or sad, pleased or angry,

The Way has no place to settle.
Love and desire: still them!
Folly and disturbance: correct them!
Do not push it! do not pull it!
Good fortune will naturally return to you,
And that Way will naturally come to you
So you can rely on and take counsel from it.
If you are tranquil then you will attain it;
If you are agitated then you will lose it.

Twenty-six

That mysterious vital energy within the mind:
One moment it arrives, the next it departs.
So fine, there is nothing within it;
So vast, there is nothing outside it.
We lose it
Because of the harm caused by mental agitation.
When the mind can hold on to tranquility,
The Way will become naturally stabilized.
For people who have attained the Way
It permeates their pores and saturates their hair.
Within their chest, they remain unvanquished.
[Follow] this Way of restricting sense-desires
And the myriad things will not cause you harm.

Reference: http://www.stillness.com/tao/neiyeh.txt
Book: Harold D. Roth Original Tao: Inward Training (Nei-yeh) and
the Foundations of Taoist Mysticism

Taiji Master

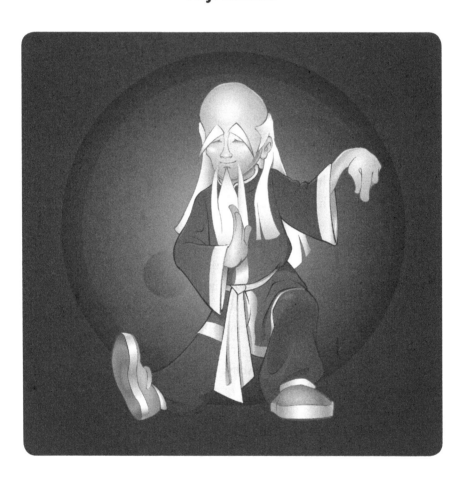

Conclusion: Final Observations

One must understand that Taijiquan is a real martial art that takes a lot of practice, perseverance and study in order to reach a high level. Taijiquan is the art of self-cultivation and is an ultimate art because it reaches beyond the idea of a martial art and becomes a lifelong practice into cultivation and the expansion of consciousness. Taijiquan changes your mind and body and energy and raises the art to one of higher art for those who are dedicated to its practice. One can reach higher levels if one understands that there is a higher level. I do not worry about the level, just practice the art and strive to perfect my practice. This requires not only doing forms, but also understanding the essence of Taijiquan and how to incorporate the essence into my practice.

The wonders of Taijiquan is there but remember the mountain of attainment, there is always another mountain to climb which makes me smile because I realize like the mind we cannot see the end. Just like the Dao it is everywhere we are. We just have to experience and enjoy it. As one grows the joy is in the journey and the practice, and then the sharing.

The joy of the practice is when one sees progress and senses the changes and growth that is realized from the art. Taijiquan is a complete martial art system and a true Chinese Treasure. As more and more people are learning Taiji one hopes they learn the art of Taiji and not just the basic forms of Taiji but if that is all you learn enjoy your practice. I realize the promise of a high art practice is dedication to perfection but I practice unafraid to achieve the high bar raised by the Masters who have tread the path before me, and know the higher goal is in front of me and I can reach out and touch it for it is there for all who would seek to know they can achieve it.

The traditional will always show one the way since the ancestors came before us and left evidence in the way of classics to guide us in the way.

Modern thought approaches the scientific but remember all cannot be measured in the lab. Just like everyone is not the same and the practice is individual. Remember either you believe or you do not does not change the truth or the obvious or the obscure. Armed with the classics, a good teacher and an inner guidance will help you arrive not only at the inner door but to the upper chamber of mastery so do not give up and know success is in your future. If we only cultivate our consciousness, become healthy, achieve longevity and become universal we have achieved our goal. Cultivate excellence and the ultimate art of Taijiquan will be a goal achieved. Know that the more you practice the deeper and higher art will be revealed. So stay on the path, keep learning, practicing, being patient, and perservering, all for art's sake!

About the Author

George writes to assist with the spreading of knowledge and light to all who seek to educate themselves on a variety of levels. This new book on Mastering Taijiquan is vital for all those who seek to study and practice the wonderous art where there is a need for the sharing of information and wisdom so that the blind will not lead the blind down the wrong path are ring around the merry-go-round. There is a serious need to share experiences and knowledge amongst practicitioners and seekers of the art of Taijiquan. George is a practitioner and Teacher of Chinese internal martial arts. George Samuels, is an enlightened realized Spiritual Master, Guide, Teacher, Healer, Spiritual Coach, Author and Poet, and he is here to teach and help heal those who seek answers and want to learn in order to help others. Master George has been providing Light, spiritual wisdom, healing, coaching, and spiritual guidance for thousands of people throughout the USA and other countries for more than 30 years. He continues to and is currently helping and healing all who contact him and are seeking Light on the Path. George provides Insight, Readings, Spiritual Counseling, Coaching and Training Classes on every level In-person or long distance and includes Qigong Healing, Tai Chi Gong and Internal Boxing. Below is a brief profile of his study and research into Martial Arts.

George is a lifetime member of the USAWKF (United States Wushu and Kungfu Federation), and member of American Chen Federation. George has studied various styles of martial arts that include Japanese Goju Ru style Karate for many years and Chinese martial arts. This also includes various styles of Yang Style Taiji Chuan modern styles such as 24, 42, and 37; Yang Ban Hao style 108 forms; Chung Style 108 forms; Chen Style Lao Jia and Xin Jia long forms including cannon fist forms; Liu He Ba Fa (6 harmonies 8 methods Water Style Boxing); 72 Closed Hands part of Swimming Dragon Chuan. This includes various weapons including Jian and Dao, Fan, Staff. George has competed in numerous major tournaments in America, Hong Kong and China and has won numerous gold, silver and bronze medals.

George has also been a tournament Judge for various National American, Japanese and Chinese Martial Arts Tournaments. Liu Xiao Lin's (Omei) Tournament in Virginia

I have been a judge for Push Hands tournament for Wu Shen Tao School in Maryland

Judge for Tournaments in Houston Texas for Jung Chian 's Traditional Tournaments

Tournament Judge for San Diego Martial Arts Tournaments from 2009 to present. George has also taught Yang and Chen style Taiji Chuan in Maryland, Virginia, and Florida and awarded Teacher and Coach certification in America for Taiji Chuan, and qualified to teach in China.

George is a Master Healer and Master Teacher and have also studied in the US and in China: Qigong, Dim Mak and Chi Healing. He has taught Self Defense Techniques, Healing and Chi Kung (Qigong) for several years to private and public students and continues to help and advise those who cross his path. George has studied with a variety of Grandmasters and Master Teachers of which a few is mentioned below such as Grand Master Lu Xiao Lin, Grand Master Yu Yin Sen, Grand Master Chen Xiaowang, Grand master Chen Zheng Lei, Grand Master

Liu Shr Bao, Grand Master Yu AnRen, Master Yu Xiao Lin, Master George Xu, Master Chen Song-Tso.

My Websites

www.spirituallifesource.com
www.taijigonghealinginstitute.com
www.gsamuelsbooksandart.com

Glossary of Terms

Dantian, dan t'ian, dan tien or tan t'ien is loosely translated as "elixir field", "sea of Qi", or simply "energy center".

Fa jin, fajin, or fa chin (fā jìn, 發勁) is a term used in some Chinese martial arts, particularly the neijia (internal) martial arts, such as Xingyiquan,

Pushing hands or is the name for two-person training routines practiced in internal Chinese martial arts such as Baguazhang, Xingyiquan, T'ai chi ch'uan (Taijiquan), Liuhebafa, Ch'uan Fa, and Yiquan.

Yin & yang, which are often shortened to "yin-yang" or "yin yang", are concepts used to describe how apparently opposite or contrary forces are actually complementary,

Kung fu/Kungfu or Gung fu/Gongfu (功夫, Pinyin: gōngfu) is a Chinese term referring to any study, learning, or practice that requires patience, energy, and time to complete, often used in the West to refer to Chinese martial arts.

Zhanzhuang, literally: "standing like a post", is a training method often practiced by students of neijia (internal kung fu), such as Xing Yi Quan, Bagua Zhang and Taiji Quan.

Qi (more precisely qì, also chi, ch'i or ki) is an active principle forming part of any living thing. *Qi* is frequently translated as "natural energy", "life force", or "energy flow". *Qi* is the central underlying principle in traditional Chinese medicine and martial arts.

The term **wushu** is Chinese for "martial arts" (武 "Wu" = military or martial, 术 "Shu" = art). In contemporary times, wushu has become an international sport

Shifu (Mandarin Chinese) is an accomplished teacher who oversees apprentices in certain traditions and philosophies. It is written with the Chinese characters: 師傅and師父. The character師means "teacher"

Jīng (Chinese: 精; Wade-Giles: ching¹) is the Chinese word for "essence"

Nèijiā (Chinese: 內家; literally: "internal school") is a term in Chinese martial arts, grouping those styles that practice nèijìng (Chinese: 內勁; literally: "internal strength"), usually translated as internal martial arts, occupied with spiritual, mental or Qi-related aspects,

Neigong, also spelled *nei kung, neigung,* or *nae gong,* refers to any of a set of Chinese breathing, meditation and spiritual practice disciplines associated with Daoism and especially the Chinese martial arts. Neigong practice is normally associated with the so-called "soft style", "internal" or neijia內家Chinese martial arts,

External style (Chinese: 外家; pinyin: *wàijiā*; literally: "external family") are often associated with Chinese martial arts. They are characterized by fast and explosive movements and a focus on physical strength and agility.

An - Push, Press, Pressing, Stamping (an4) 按 (TX) One of the 13 Postures of Taijiquan.

An Jin - **Hidden Power**

Ao Bu - Twisted Stance, Reverse Stance 拗步 A stance in which the opposite foot and hand are forward, e.g., right foot and left hand are in front of the left foot and right hand.

Ba Gua - Eight Trigrams (*I Ching*)

Breath, Energy, Life Force - *Chi, Qi* 氣

Brush Knee and Twist Step - *Lou Xi Ao Bu* 搂膝拗步 [#10, 17, 25, 44,] (T)

Book of Changes – Yi (*I*) *Ching* (Jing)

Breath and Energy Training Work - ***Qigong, Chi Kung***

Broadsword *(Dao*

Breathing Exercises - *Nei Gong, Nei Kung* 內功

Brush Knee and Twist Step - *Lou Zi Ao Bu*

Bu - Step, Stepping 步 (bù)

Cai - Pluck, Pick

Central Equilibrium - *Zhong Ding*

Chi - Breath, Energy, Life Force 氣

Chi Kung, *Qigong* - Energy and Breath Training Work 氣功

Chen Family Style Taijiquan 陈氏 太极拳

Close, Combine, Unite, Join - *He* 合

Close Hands, Closing Hands - *He Shou* 合手

Cloud Hands - *Yun Shou* 云手

Crossing - *Héng* 橫

Commencing Form - *Qi Shi*

Da - Strike, Striking

Dan Bian [*dan1 bian1*] - Single Whip 单鞭

Dao De Jing, *Tao Te Ching* - "Book of the Way and Its Virture" by Lao Tzu 道德經

Dao Nian Hou [*dao4 nian3 hou2*] - Step Back and Repulse Monkey 倒撵猴

Down - Xia

Eight Energies of Taijiquan: *Peng* (Ward Off), *Lu* (Rollback), *Ji* (Press), *An* (Push), *Cai* (Pluck) *Lie* (Rend), *Kao* (Shoulder Stroke), and *Zhou* (Elbow).

Eight Trigrams - *Ba Gua*

Elbow - *Zhou*

Embrace Tiger, Push Mountain - *Bao Hu Tui Shan* 抱虎归山

Energy, Breath, Life Force - *Qi, Chi* 氣

Energy and Breath Training Work - *Qigong, Chi Kung* 氣功

Fair Lady Works the Shuttles - *Yu Nu Chuan Suo* 玉女穿梭

Fan Through the Back - *Shan Tong Bei* 扇通背

Fist Under Elbow - *Zhou Di Kan Quan, Zhou Di Kan Chui* 肘底捶

Flowing Steps Taijiquan Form - *Huo Bu Jia Taijiquan*

Form, Style, Type, Pattern, Rule - *Shi* 式

Forms, Solo Forms or Solo Routines - *Taolu* 套路

Gao Hu Gui Shuan - Embrace Tiger, Push Mountain 抱虎归山

Gao Shi - High Stance or Posture

Gao Tan Ma - High Pat on Horse 高探马

Golden Rooster Stands on One Leg - *Jin Ji Du Li* 金鸡独立

Gong - An Accomplishment or Skill Attained from Effort, Practice, Hard Work, Discipline

Grand Ultimate Boxing - ***Taijiquan***

Guitar - *Pi Pa*

Hands, Hands - *Shou*

He - Close 合 (he2)

He Shou - Close Hands 合手 (T)

High Pat on Horse - *Gao Tan Ma* 高探马

Hidden Power - *An Jin*

Hsing I Chuan - Mind/Form Boxing, Form Intention, Shape Will, Mind/Will Boxing 形意拳

I Ching - Book of Changes

Internal Martial Arts - *Nei Jia Quan*

Jade Girl Working with Shuttles - *Yu Nu Chuan Suo* 玉女穿梭

Ji - Press, Squeeze

JIan, Chien, Gim - Sword (Straight) 劍

Jian Bu Da Chui - Step Forward, Punch Low 进步栽锤

Jin Ji Du Li - Golden Rooster Stands on One Leg 金鸡独立

Kai 开 - Open

Kai Shou - Open Hands, Opening Hands 开手 (開手)

Kao - Shoulder Stroke, Leaning

Lan Zha Yi - Leisurely Tying Clothes, Lazily Tucking in Coat, Tuck in Robes 懒扎衣 (lǎn zhā yī)

Lazily Tying Clothes - *Lan Zha Yi* 懒扎衣

Lìe - Rend

Lift, Lifting - *Ti* 提

Li Jin, Li Qi, Li - Muscular Power

Lu - Rollback, Pull

Muscular Power - *Li Qi* or *Jin*

Nei Gong, Nei Kung - Breathing Exercises 内功

Nei Jia Quan - Internal Martial Arts, IMA, Chinese Taoist Influenced Martial Arts

No Extremity, Undifferentiated, Emptiness, Chaos - *Wuji*

Open - *Kai* 开

Opening Hands - *Kai Shou*

Pào - Pounding, Pound 炮

Parting the Wild Horse's Mane - Ye Ma Fen Zong

Peng - Ward Off, Blocking

Pi Pa - Lute, Guitar

Pluck - *Cai*

Press - *Ji*

Pressing, Stamping - *An*

Push, Press, Control, Restrain - *An* 按

Pushing Hands - *T'ui Shou* 推手

Qi - Energy, Life Force, Power, Aliveness

Qi - Starting, Rise, Raise Up (qǐ) 起

Qi Jin - Vigorously, Energetically, Enthusiastically 起勁 (qǐ jÌn)

Qi Li, *Li Qi, Li Jin - Muscular Power*

Qigong, Chi Kung - Energy and Breath Training Work 氣功

Qi Shi - Commencing Form

Relaxation, Openness, Calm Awareness - *Song, Sung*

Rend - *Lìe*

Right Hand - You Shou

Rollback - *Lu*

Ru Feng Si Bi [*ru2 feng1 si4 bi4*] - Apparent Close Up, Appearing to Seal and Close, Apparent Close 如封似闭

San Ti - Three Essentials, Trinity Posture (Heaven, Man, Earth) in Sun's *Xing I Quan*

San Ti_Shi - Three Essentials Form, Trinity Posture (Heaven, Man, Earth) in Sun's *Xing I Quan,* the basic Xing I Quan posture

Shan Tong Bei - Fan Through the Back 扇通背

Shi - Style, Type, Form, Pattern, Rule *(*shì, shi4*)* 式

Shoulder Stroke - *Kao*

Single Whip - *Dan Bian* 单鞭

Song, Sung - Relaxation, Letting Go of Unnecessary Tension

Splitting, Split, Split Like an Axe - *Pī* 劈

Step, Stepping - *Bu* 步 (bù)

Straight and Centered - *Zhong Zheng*

Sung - Relaxation, Openness, Calm Awareness

Sword (Straight) - *JIan, Chien, Gim* 劍

T'ai Chi Ch'uan, *Taijiquan* - Grand Ultimate Boxing, Boundless Fist 太极拳

T'ai Chi, Taiji Symbol, Ying/Yang Symbol - *Taijitu* or *T'ai Chi T'u* 太極圖

Taiji - Grand Ultimate, the Synergy of Yin and Yan

Tai Ji Quan, Taijiquan, T'ai Chi Ch'uan 太极拳

Taijiquan - Grand Ultimate Boxing, Boundless Fist

Te (dě)

n.

1. In Taoism, the power through which the Tao is made manifest or is actualized.
2. In Confucianism, the virtuous moral strength embodied in wise people, upon which they rely in times of distress.

T'ai Chi T'u or Taijitu - Taiji Symbol, Ying/Yang Symbol 太極圖

Tao Te Ching, *Dao De Jing* - "Book of the Way and Its Virture" by Lao Tzu 道德經

Taolu - Forms, Solo Forms or Solo Routines 套路

Trinity Posture (Heaven, Man, Earth) - *San Ti Shi*

Tuck in Robes - *Lan Zha Yi* 懶扎衣

T'ui Shou - Pushing Hands 推手

Tui Bu Shan Zhang - Back Step and Wave Palms

Twist Step, Brush Knee and Push, Left Side - *Zuo Lou Xi Ao Bu* 左搂膝拗步

Tying Back the Coat, Tuck in Robes - *Lan Zha Yi*

Vigorously, Energetically, Enthusiastically - *Qi Jin* 起勁 (qǐ jÌn)

Ward Off - *Peng*

Wave Hands Like Clouds - *Yun Shou* 云手

Whip - Single - *Dan Bian* 单鞭

White Crane Spreads Wings - *Bai He Liang Chi* 白鹤凉翅

White Swan (Goose, Crane) Spreads Its Wings - *Bai He Liang Chi* 白鹤凉翅

Wuji - No Extremity, Stillness and Quiet, Without Characteristics, Chaos, Emptiness,

Wuji - Taiji - Opening Movement, Commencement

Research materials and Additional Reading

Tai Chi Classics

The classic texts below trace the philosophy of Tai Chi Chuan, which advises not resisting force but using it to your own advantage.

T'AI CHI CH'UAN CHING Attributed to Chang San-feng

THE TREATISE ON T'AI CHI CH'UAN Attributed to Wang Tsung-yueh [Wang Zongyue]

EXPOSITIONS OF INSIGHTS INTO THE PRACTICE OF THE THIRTEEN POSTURES by Wu Yu-hsiang (Wu Yuxian)

SONG OF THE THIRTEEN POSTURES Unknown Author

SONGS OF THE EIGHT POSTURES Attributed to T'an Meng- hsienas

SONG OF PUSH HANDS Unknown Author

FIVE CHARACTER SECRET by Li I-yu

ESSENTIALS OF THE PRACTICE OF THE FORM AND PUSH-HANDS by Li I-yu

YANG'S TEN IMPORTANT POINTS by Yang Cheng-fu

Wikipedia, Article on T'ai chi ch'uan

Approaching Core Principles. By Sam Masich.

Cheng Man-Ch'ing (1901-1975) Six Excellances

Chinese Philosophy and Tai Chi Chuan. By Dan Docherty.

Clarifying the Meaning of Peng Energy. By Hiu Chee Fatt. *T'ai Chi*, April, 2002, Volume 26

The Complete Book of Tai Chi Chuan: A Comprehensive Guide to the Principles and Practice. By Wong, Kiew Kit

The Essence of T'ai Chi Ch'uan: The Literary Tradition. Translated and edited by Benjamin Pang Jeng Lo; Martin Inn, Robert Amacker, and Susan Foe. Berkeley, California, North Atlantic Books

Expositions of Insights Into the Practice of the Thirteen Postures. By Wu, Yu-hsiang. Paraphrased by Lee N. Scheele.

Expositions of Insights Into the Practice of the Thirteen Postures. By Wu, Yu-hsiang (Wu Yuxian) 1812-1880

Five Steps: Meditative Sensation Walking. By Paul Crompton. Midpoint Trade Books, 1999

Mental Elucidation of the Thirteen Postures By Wu Yu Xiang.

Rooting: The Secret of Getting Power from the Earth. By Gaofei Yan and James Cravens.

Songs of the Eight Postures. Attributed to T'an, Meng-hsien. As researched by Lee N. Scheele.

T'ai Chi Classics. By Waysun Liao.

Tai Chi 13 Postures. By Zhang Yun

 Tai Chi Touchstones: Yang Family Secret Transmissions. Translation, commentary and editing by Douglas Wile.

The Tao of T'ai-Chi Ch'uan: Way to Rejuvenation. By Jou, Tsung, Hwa.

Expositions of Insights Into the Practice of the Thirteen Postures. By Wu, Yu-hsiang. Paraphrased by Lee N. Scheele.

Printed in the United States
By Bookmasters